# Praise fo

This book is so powerful. It gave me insight to all the things that Sandy and Rick went through together. It has helped both my husband and I to process all the feelings we encountered (Do I have cancer? and How this will change everything in our lives?) before, during and after my visit to Stanford to get the breast exam I needed when I noticed a change in my breast. Learning about what Sandy went through and felt brought out feelings so strong that it was cathartic for me. I was able to better understand the emotions and feelings I was going through, realizing that they were real and I shouldn't just forget about them, and how they effected me physically, emotionally, and spiritually. Get two copies of this book—one for you and one to give to a friend who will really need it.
—*Kelly V*

The healing that occurs throughout this book is clearly a by-product of the biblical concept of laying on of hands. This is a gift from God. Energy is an essential part of all of life. The Craniosacral process is nothing new under the sun, it's right in the Bible. It's a gift given to us. How beautiful to witness the healing power.
—*Linda E*

Sandy bravely shares her life and journey through cancer and treatment with a mix of delightful stories and gut wrenching emotion. I have only experienced cancer as a friend and sister. My brother, Dave, was diagnosed with colon cancer nearly five years ago, and as I read about Sandy's trials I wondered about him. Would the same, amazing post-chemo treatment have helped him? Reading *Life after Chemo* has broadened my understanding of both the medical and spiritual journeys that Sandy and many others have endured.
—*Sue Y.*

This is more than just a human interest story. It is a spiritual journey into the depths of ones soul. It is God's grace in the midst of the adversity of cancer. This book made me think deeply of where the 'manna' is hiding in my life. You'll find it both educational and inspiring!
—*Chad S.*

This is one of the best books I've ever read. If I ever had cancer, it would be the first book I would want to read. My friends and relatives will all be getting a copy for Christmas. Two thumbs up!!
—*Fred T.*

# Life after Chemo

Complete Physical and Emotional Healing
from Cancer Is Possible

By
Sandy Howard

*Printed in the United States of America*

Sandy Howard
P.O. Box 1214
Los Banos, California 93635
lifeafterchemo@aol.com

Production Services:
Word Dancer Press, Sanger, Ca. 93657 (800) 497-4909


Published in association with and distributed by:
Loose Change Publications, 936 6th Street, Los Banos, CA 93635
(209) 826-3797 email nco4242@sbcglobal.net

To my parents, you are awesome. Thanks for blessing me with the beautiful gift of a healthy and happy childhood.

To our beautiful kids, Joel, Kate, Mallory, and Bryce. You are the bright lights in our lives.

And to Rick, my Knight in Shining Armor, my best friend; your amazing love soothes, energizes, and refreshes me daily, thank you, my love.

I couldn't have done it without you.

---

"You, the individual, can do more for your health and well-being than any doctor, any hospital, any drug, and any exotic medical device."

—Joseph Califano

---

*God resists the proud, but gives grace to the humble. Therefore humble yourselves under the mighty hand of God, that He may exalt you IN DUE TIME, casting all your cares upon Him, for He loves and cares for you. I Peter 5: 6&7*

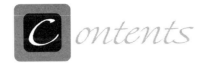

# Contents

*1*

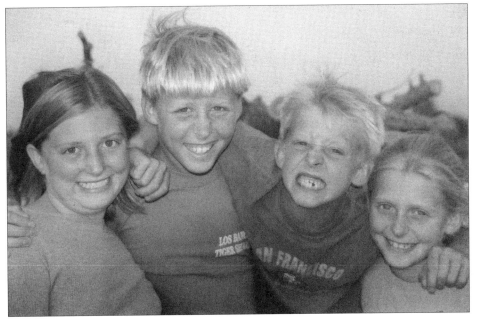

*My beautiful kids: Kate, Joel, Bryce, and Mallory*

# Blindsided

"Tell me about your children," the nurse said as she began to empty the huge tube of red liquid into my IV. The tears welled up; I couldn't speak. My kids. My four precious kids. Would I live to see them grow up? Would I be there for their weddings? Know my grandchildren, their spouses? Joel, my oldest at 14. How was God going to use his life? Would he go into the ministry that he seemed so gifted for? How would He use precious Kate? Would Mallory become the actress she dreamed of becoming? Where would God lead our Bryce? The knot in my throat was choking me; I was horrified at the events that had so recently unfolded. Watching the fluid flow in my arm, I thought, "Lord, I'm in the best shape of my life, I eat right, I love and worship you, why are you allowing this? I trust you, but I'm having some doubts here about what's happening. Is this really your plan?"

Two weeks earlier, I had buzzed over to the doctor's for my annual pap smear. I was so healthy and happy; my life was so blessed. Four wonderful kids and Rick, my amazing husband of 16 years. I'd have a quick exam and I'd be back on the road.

But during the exam of my left breast, Dr. Wang paused and palpated the same area again…and again. I couldn't even ask. My stomach started to tingle. I just watched the concern etched on his face. Finally, "Have you ever felt this? No, leave your arm up over your head; now feel." Wham, a hard spot the size and shape of my pointer finger. Like a pop-up book, when I put my arm down it went away. When I raised my arm, it popped out.

"No, I've never checked myself with my arm up." Aside from cursory exams in the shower, I was certainly not a role model when it came to breast exams. Why check myself? It would never happen to me. I had a healthy diet, exercised, no family history of breast cancer. I had nursed my four babies, a factor that statistically lowers the odds for breast cancer, and I had only used the pill for two years at the beginning of our marriage. I certainly was no candidate for cancer. But this huge lump. I felt it again. Yeah, it definitely was there. And I knew it was cancer. My chest felt like a huge hollow cave. I had to concentrate to breathe. I knew God was in control, but suddenly I felt like all the pieces of my neat and tidy life had been tossed up in the air.

"You need to make an appointment for an x-ray and a follow-up appointment for two weeks."

"Two weeks? Wait for two weeks to find out for sure?" The notion seemed insane. I cried as I drove home. I cried for my kids, for my husband, my family, myself. I felt as if I was putting them on a roller coaster ride without the lap bar. Why did God let this happen to *me*?

On the other hand, in a weird way, in the very back of my mind, it was a relief to know what my *trauma* would be. I mean, everyone has to go through some difficulty in their lives, right? Maybe if I just got through this and endured with some dignity, we would pass the stress test and not have any more trials. I had lived with the dread of something bad happening to one of our kids. It was the mentality of My life is so good, I wonder when something is going to happen. I feared one of my kids dying, or worse, having to live the rest of their lives in a wheelchair. I had worked as a nurse at a Muscular Dystrophy camp one summer. The struggles those beautiful children endured had made a deep impression on me. Worse still was the thought that something might happen to my precious husband, Rick. I couldn't even entertain the thought of life without him or seeing him in pain. So this was it, this was to be my challenge. At least it was me and not one of them. I would much rather suffer, than see one of them hurting. My life had been so wonderful and blessed to this point. I didn't know that day that I would eventually come to view cancer as one of the greatest blessings in my life.

My husband is the most practical and logical man I know. A successful businessman, his ideals have served him well. And when it is said that opposites attract, we can be a case study. So, when I told Rick that we'd have to wait two weeks he said, "What? Two weeks? If we took you to the vet, we'd get better service than that! There's no way we wait two weeks to read an x-ray."

Through a friend of a friend, I was put in contact with the Stanford Breast Center. Fortunately Stanford was only a couple hours' drive from our home. I called on Thursday and had an appointment for the following Tuesday. I was operating in stealth mode. I didn't want the kids to worry, but I desperately needed the prayer of friends. Rick's tactic was to say nothing to anyone until we knew for sure, but I felt like a volcano ready to blow.

Saturday at our kids' swim meet, I pulled my closest friends aside and shared my news. It was such a relief to get it off my chest, but at the same time I felt guilty burdening them with my *secret.* They offered the encouragement and support I craved. Swim meets last all day, and this meet was brutally long. I had a knot in my stomach. I was an inch from tears, but thankfully I was surrounded by friends.

Swim team has its own unique culture. We had ventured into the world of swimming when Joel, our oldest, was nine, and Bryce, the youngest was four. We were looking for a sport that allowed all the kids to practice at the same place and at the same time. The kids had been involved in soccer, basketball, and little league. And with each kid's different practice and game time, the schedule was crazy. Most of our friends were also on the swim team, so the Saturday meets were one big party. We packed in ice chests and chairs and hung out under shade canopies.

The day was usually quite relaxing. Bryce brought his little John Deere pedal tractor and raced around the park—he was entertained and out of our hair. The girls played with their friends and had fun in their races, while Joel actually took the sport quite seriously. He turned out to be a natural; he won races from day one. Rick's highlight of the meet, besides cheering on his cute kids, became the "Twitchell." Mrs. Twitchell was the head of our hospitality team.

These wonderful ladies, who took their jobs quite seriously, served drinks and snacks to the timers and other event workers throughout the hot day. Mrs. Twitchell raised the bar to a new level when she brought in her Vitameataveggiemiester, one of those huge blenders that could pulverize your hand in less than three seconds if you happened to slip while dropping in the strawberries. When she cranked that baby up the first time, heads swiveled. What was going on in the hospitality tent? The roar was deafening. She blended Gatorade mix and ice, a painfully simple combination, but on a hot day people would kill to get their hands on one of those drinks. Suddenly those volunteer positions that were hard to fill had waiting lists. "Can I time for the next shift?" You see, the only way to qualify for a "Twitchell" was to be volunteering your time to the team. They just tasted like heaven. Rick didn't work, he just befriended Mrs. Twitchell, and every time the Vitameataveggiemiester roared, he jumped up and took a walk. Mrs. Twitchell would greet him with a smile and a fresh drink, and he would smugly saunter around the pool deck, slowly sipping the latest concoction.

After the swim meet, we headed down to our neighbor's house for a barbecue. The Martins were remodeling their backyard and planning to add a pool. A friend who had experienced breast cancer was at the party. We quietly discussed how the appointment Tuesday would probably unfold. She explained all the current procedures: lumpectomy, mastectomy, rebuild the breast during the surgery, or wait until later for the Take-your-fat-stomach-and-shove-it-into-the-space-your-boob-used-to-be technique. There were so many different treatments and options. I knew this was happening fast, and I wanted to be prepared when I got there. No more surprises.

That night, lying in bed, I gave Rick a quick rundown on what I had learned my options might be. After the rundown, I asked Rick for his opinion. "I wonder where the Martins are going to put their pool..."

I was amazed, shocked, I was totally hurt. I knew he loved me, he was a wonderful man and husband, but he was somehow totally ignoring the fact that his wife had cancer. What was going on? I knew trauma either tore families apart or brought them together. Was this how it happened? Was he going to pull away from me? I lay awake in fear that night. What was happening to my husband? What was happening to me?

The message on the answering machine Monday sent shockwaves through my body. "Hello, this is the oncology breast specialty clinic calling to confirm an appointment for Sandy tomorrow at 12:00." My heart stopped. What if my kids heard that message? Would they know what *oncology* meant? I was desperate to protect them as long as possible—at least until we knew what was going on and could explain everything calmly and answer all their questions. I shut the office door and quickly called the clinic back to confirm my appointment. I asked the receptionist to make a note not to mention the word Stanford or oncology on any further messages. It was worth a try.

Stanford is big and efficient; it is also a teaching hospital. Doctors are always accompanied by residents, mutts, as we came to know and tolerate them. Releases signed prior to all appointments warn that Stanford is a teaching institution and that residents will be accompanying the doctors. "No problem," I thought. "After all, I was a student nurse once too…"

I was a cold stone, frozen on the exam table. Rick sat in the corner attempting chitchat. I was just too nervous to participate. Dr. Denis entered; he was a tall, thin, serious-looking man. This guy probably does calculus problems before bed for relaxation. A mutt stood by his side. After introductions, he got right to business. "Oh, you found a lump? Which breast? May I see it please?"

I lay back, that crackling tissue under me sounded like a thousand newspapers being wadded up. I nervously pulled down my gown. He didn't waste any time beginning the exam. He was a master at the poker face. I stared up at him intently and caught the sudden squint in his eyes when he got to my lump. My heart stopped. I willed him to say, "Oh, that's nothing! Who referred you here, anyway?" He clearly was not going to fulfill my greatest desire. Instead, I could see his concern deepen.

He palpated, and palpated again. A little measuring stick was whisked out from his lab coat pocket to measure the area. It was the length and width of my middle finger. I already knew. "Do you mind if Dr. X palpates this area?"

"No, I just want to go home," I thought, but replied, "Sure…" More fingers lightly drumming my breast. There was clearly a technique for this. It interestingly involved rapid finger movement, somewhat like typing one hundred words per minute on the same line of the keyboard while slowly climbing from the base of the breast to the top. I wondered how many breasts this guy had felt. Was I just another body? Was he fighting to disassociate me from sexual thoughts? Well, at least my mind was working… it's just what you think about while strange men feel your breast. I blinked as Dr. X stepped back from the exam table.

"Now if you'll sit up, Mrs. Howard." I pulled my gown back on and quickly popped up, relieved to have that part of the exam over. "Now take both arms out of the gown and sit up nice and straight." Oh great, there was more. Sit here with my gown totally off? They were serious. I was looking for them to crack a smile. Surely they were joking. No, they definitely weren't. I considered passing on this round. It seemed like a case of serious overexposure, but I was in no position to question. I needed their help. I complied. I sat up nice and straight while they took a few paces back, and with their hands on their chins, seriously speculated my chest.

"Hold your arms up straight." More speculation. I was staring at them, trying to read their thoughts without any success. "OK, now hold your arms straight out from your side, elbows bent, fists toward the ceiling." It took me a minute to process that one. OK, they want to see me flex. More thoughtful speculation. They bent forward at the waist a bit, trying to get a better look. I couldn't resist tightening my fists and flexing my biceps a bit. At least my vanity's still intact. Finally, I was asked to put my gown back on. I was relieved to be done but dreaded what he would say. It was definitely something he wanted to explore; in fact, an ultrasound the following day was recommended. My stomach contracted.

We thought it would be easier to have Rick stay home with the kids the next day to maintain some sense of normalcy. This trip would be strictly a test, in and out, with no new information given. My cycling buddy Dana went with me. Dana and I were into biking, and since we had tried a couple of short triathlons the previous year, I was shocked to see a poster of a woman competing in a triathlon on the procedure room wall. The woman in the poster had a very determined look on her face. I found it hugely inspiring. I also found it comforting that there would be a triathlon poster at this time and in this place. God was reassuring me, supporting me. I whispered thanks. The doctor looked very fit, so I asked her what she did for workouts.

"I cycle," she replied.

"Like a road bike?" I was so amazed. What were the odds? "Yeah," her assistant chimed in, "she does century rides and double century rides!" I shook my head in amazement. Dana and I had done a century ride last year, also! I had an instant friend here, a comrade. Whatever she said, I trusted. I know their fitness and sport of choice did not reflect their medical ability; nonetheless, I felt a total peace and comfort.

"I've done a couple of short triathlons myself," the technician Jenn chimed in.

"OK, so here I am, surrounded by a picture of a triathlete; my doctor and nurse are triathletes and bikers. I hear you, Lord. You are here with me, aren't you?" The four of us yakked bikes the rest of the procedure. I was so thankful to be in good hands.

A biopsy was scheduled for the following day. The kids still believed I was taking vacation days, a fun day in the city. My friend Laura accompanied me for this trip. I dreaded it. I felt like a heavy weight was on my chest. "Why me? Why not me? Thank you, Lord, for this. In everything I must give thanks. I know you are in control. You know everything – if I could just back up and choose a different tack – just change course a little and swerve off this cancer track, I would sure love to do it. I don't want to drink from this cup, Lord, but I promise to deal with it faithfully leaning on you. So bring it on, Lord, if this is how it's supposed to be."

We had to wait five days for the final report. "It's tough, fibrous tissue which might be good news," the doctor encouraged after the biopsy. "Go home and relax and think positive."

I found myself looking at my breasts in the mirror. I never cared about my breasts before; now I went out of my way to find mirrors so I could look at myself. Walking past storefronts, I would gaze at my reflection. How much longer will I look like this? Friends told me I was fortunate to be endowed; I didn't care. But now I did. I cared a lot. How would our life be without breasts? How much of my femininity would be excised with my breasts, if it came to that? Since I had always taken them for granted, now I truly appreciated them for their feminine qualities. I held myself at night in bed, especially the offended site. Much like you would cradle a broken arm, I cradled my breast. It was wounded, but it was a part of me and I desperately wanted to keep it.

I got mad that night. Very, very angry. I did not want to have cancer. I didn't want anything to do with it. I didn't want my family to have to go through this trial. I didn't want to hurt my kids, my husband, my parents. I just didn't want to go down this road. I fumed around the house. I was in a major bad mood. I went to bed mad. I even started cussing out God. It felt so good to let Him have it. I woke up and picked up where I left off until I finally slowed down long enough to realize how pathetic I was. Here I was, a speck in the universe, and I had the audacity to curse the Almighty God who created me and the entire universe! I've always felt it's better to join them than fight them, so I decided it was time to get past this anger. It was still early in the morning, so I went downstairs, got on the couch with my Bible, and started looking up all the verses having to do with suffering. After flipping to a few, I landed in the book of Peter, the book of suffering. I read I Peter 5:6: "God resists the proud, but gives grace to the humble. Therefore humble yourselves under the mighty hand of God, that He may exalt you *in due time*, casting all your cares upon Him, for He loves and cares for you."

I started crying, as I was reminded of His immense love for me. He loves me more than I could ever comprehend. He knows every hair on my head. I understood I needed to humble myself under His amazing, mighty hand, and in due time, I would understand His purpose for this cancer. "Alright, Lord, I'm humbled down here and trusting you…"

We had planned a trip to hang out at our friends' beach house in Aptos for a long weekend. We decided to keep our plans and headed out the next day. My parents came along. They are fantastic grandparents, and my kids think they are just big playmates. Dad jokes around all the time and teases them. Grandma and grandpa are great fun and much loved. But this weekend, Rick and I felt like we were walking on eggshells, keeping this big, slimy secret of ours. We still didn't want to say anything, not until we had all the information. I was totally dreading telling my parents. My dad just had endured bladder cancer two years prior. Fortunately, they caught his cancer early. It was confined to his bladder and responded well to treatment. But I vividly recalled the extreme anguish my mom endured when they got the diagnosis. I didn't want her to go through that again. Dad had kept a fantastic attitude during treatment, toughing out the chemo they pushed directly into his bladder. He was now a survivor.

We spent a lot of time at the beach that weekend. We kayaked, rode the waves on our boogey boards, and relaxed with the kids. The weather was perfect. It was a wonderful distraction. "This is such a beautiful world you created, Lord. How long am I going to be in it?"

We arrived home to two messages from Dr. Denis. "Sandy, I need to talk to you."

I looked at Rick, "Uh oh." I sat down, dialed the number, and talked with Trina, one of the many wonderful people we met at the breast clinic. Rick, sitting in the chair next to me, was like a statue.

"Sandy, its lobular cancer...are you OK? . . . We need to do a PET scan and then schedule a time to meet back with Dr. Denis."

I was in a fog. I felt frozen, numb, and terrified all at once. "Is this really happening? I have cancer?"

Rick, still not reacting, "Let's just wait until we get all the information."

Renee, a cycling buddy, accompanied me to the PET scan. We took our bikes. The coolest thing about the Palo Alto area is the number of serious bikers cruising around on gorgeous bikes. I was amazed. After the PET scan, we rode to Hudart Park and up along Skyline Drive. It was an incredibly beautiful ride in the pine trees, with an amazing view. It was a weekday, and there were so many riders in spandex, we felt like we were at a sponsored event. I enjoyed every moment of every push of the pedal. I felt healthy and strong. "I don't know what my future holds, Lord, but I trust you."

The appointment with Dr. Denis was two days away. He would review all the test results and give us the final prognosis and treatment recommendations. Rick and I had previously made reservations to spend the weekend in Monterey, a beautiful, serene, coastal town. We decided to keep those reservations and head over to the coast after our appointment.

Rick had found an old stove in the barn of a recently purchased property, and I was stunned to see him loading the stove into the back of the truck. "What are you doing?" I whispered in amazement as he cinched down the ropes. "I told Ada I'd bring this stove over to their beach house. Since we're heading that way, it'll be a good chance to drop it off."

I was stunned. I thought, "I have cancer; I might be dying right now, and you're concerned about this old stove?" I couldn't fathom his insensitivity, his seemingly uncaring attitude.

"We'll have to drive a little slower, but that won't be a problem."

"Yes, that certainly is the least of our problems," I thought, as I climbed into the truck. I felt as if I were driving to my funeral as we headed over the hill toward Stanford. Rick, on the other hand, was carrying the conversation with light chatter. "Doesn't he get it?" I thought. "Doesn't he care?"

By the time we got to the hospital, I was certain he didn't care if I had cancer or not. It apparently was just a blip on his screen. He greeted the nurses and Dr. Denis in his usual, friendly manner as I sat stone cold on the examining table. After another cursory exam, Dr. Denis hit us with the final report. "Cancer. . . splash pattern. . .currently inoperable. . .might not get it all. . .lymph involvement. . .good chance for five-year survival. . ." he droned on but I didn't hear. I felt like someone had injected my body with Novocain and was beating me with a baseball bat. I couldn't talk, move, or react. Rick, on the other hand, was asking questions, good questions, clarifying the report. "We want you to meet with the tumor board next week to determine your treatment options. Any other questions?" He turned and walked out of the room. Rick got up from the chair and came over to me. He put his arms around me and then broke into huge, gasping sobs. We both cried and held each other. Time stood still. Our world stopped. It was worse than either of us imagined. In my lymph gland! There's no way! Five years to live? It just couldn't be.

And I finally understood. The pool, the stove, Rick had been in total denial these last two weeks. It wasn't until this moment that he let himself finally believe the truth.

Trina, the darling Irish nurse, came in to schedule the tumor board appointment and then quietly excused herself. Sometime later, she came back. I remember thinking I would hate to have her job, but I was so thankful someone with her compassion and gentle touch was willing to work in this place. After she scheduled the next appointment, we were free to go.

We stepped outside to *the stove*. There it was, lashed onto the back of the truck. Rick grasped the folly of it. "I can't believe we've got this dumb stove to deliver right now."

"Oh, it'll be good to see the Eriksons. Ada said she was going to be making dinner. I really don't feel like socializing, or eating, but maybe it'll be nice to be with friends right now." As we pulled away, I started crying again. "Five-year survival rate" kept ringing in my head. "No, this can't be. I won't die yet." As my sobbing subsided, I looked over at Rick. He was barely holding it together. We held hands as we silently drove, each of us absorbing the news and trying not to absorb the news. Then it was Rick's turn to break into sobs. I offered to drive, but no, he was going to drive . . . and sob.

By the time we got to Aptos, we were both exhausted. We entered the Eriksons' cozy home with salmon on the grill and asparagus steaming in the kitchen and knew this was where we were supposed to be. God still had a plan. We gave them a brief overview of our experience, and they set about to make us feel comfortable and loved. More time alone would have been a total disaster, both of us looking at each other trying not to cry. But with their family, we were able to talk and laugh and enjoy a couple of hours of normalcy before being swept back into the vortex of cancer. It was like a color movie that turned to slow motion black and white as we sat around their table enjoying good food and wine. We reminisced over those old stories you think you're tired of but love hearing just one more time. After we were thoroughly loved and re-energized, the stove was unloaded and we reluctantly said goodbye.

We thankfully had two days to pull ourselves together before coming home to face our kids. We had been to this same little hotel at least twenty times in our married life. It was our home away from home, our respite place. It had a pool that was always warm and big enough to swim laps, an all-you-can-eat breakfast buffet, a Jacuzzi that was always hot; I was happy; Rick was happy; we both were happy. It was just up from the beach where we could sit and soak up God's beauty, and across from a mall where we could get food and see a movie. We were set.

We flopped on the bed, got a piece of paper, and began making a list of God's blessings to us over the last sixteen years. How He had brought us together, our kids, their health, our church family, our many wonderful friends, all the properties He had put in our path for purchase. The list grew. It swelled. God was saying, "I love you guys! I'm in control! Don't be afraid! Trust me!" We laughed and cried as we grasped the magnitude of what He had brought us through and what He was about to bring us through. "Remember that time when Joel was two and he wandered off? We couldn't find him, and I just knew I was supposed to drive out to the highway. When I got there, he was standing in the middle of the road with a car stopped three feet from him?" It was a cold, foggy, morning, and there's no way a car can see my little boy on a highway. I could sense

God's angels surrounding him and the car, totally protecting him as I ran over and swooped him up. I can still remember the feel of his sweet, soft little body as I carried him back to my car.

We retold each other the story of our other angel encounter: We owned a cabin in Twain Harte, a beautifully serene mountain community. This cabin was remote, extremely remote, but we enjoyed the solitude on weekends. There was no phone, and no renters calling to complain. The air was clean. We loved this place. But the access road was ten miles of winding bumping, dirt.

The first year we owned it, we decided to head up one rainy winter day with our two-wheel drive truck. "I never had a four-wheel drive," the previous owner had confidently declared. "This road is always clear." The snowplow had clearly been through several times, but the previous week's storm had dumped so much snow, the snow piled on either side of the truck was six-feet high. Once we were off the paved road, we were committed. There was no place to turn around. Joel was about three, and Kate was a just a baby. Both were strapped in their car seats. The further down the road we went, the more scared I became. Snow began to fall, visibility decreased; the road was slippery and muddy. I knew it would be dark soon. Did we have enough gas to keep the engine running all night for heat?

We approached the one hill that had to be climbed before we could get to the cabin. The cab of the truck was silent. We slipped and slid halfway up the hill. This was definitely not working. Rick backed down the hill to give it another go. We prayed silently and began our second futile attempt up the hill. As we agonizingly ground to halt, we were stunned to see a jeep appear over the crest of the hill and drive down toward us. This was an old Willy's Jeep with four huge, chained snow tires. It ground slowly toward us. A big, burly man with a long beard climbed out and greeted Rick. "You folks need a tow?"

Yeah, we sure did. Within ten minutes, he had hooked us up with a chain, pulled us up and over the ridge, and kept on going! He pulled us the remaining distance to the cabin. We thanked him profusely, invited him in for coffee, snacks, anything he wanted. "No, thanks, I've got to go."

"Do you live around here?"

"Yes, I live just down the road."

Well, we can thank him properly when we're thawed out, we thought.

But we never got a chance to thank him again. We asked everyone in the area about the big guy with the Willy's Jeep. No one had ever seen him or heard of him. God had sent an angel to help us that day.

God had faithfully provided for us, and protected us our whole lives. Now we needed to trust Him completely. We held each other a lot that weekend.

One of the many blessings of a hick town, the small town setting I had so hugely wanted to avoid, is that, good or bad, news travels fast. I was suddenly thankful that everyone did know my business, because they were all there to offer support and encouragement. In a small town, everyone either is related to someone else, or works with or attends church with someone else. And everyone just knew. And they all responded. I was fascinated to discover that the people who responded most vigorously, even those I barely knew, were those who had previously experienced their own trauma. They already knew how comforting it was to be loved by the town.

The outpouring of love was completely staggering. On Rick's daily trek to our P.O. Box, he grew used to the daily volume of cards, cards offering encouragement, prayer, and support. Families dropped by with flowers, sometimes a single rose from someone I didn't even know very well. I received many beautiful little ceramic angels. Meals poured in, and some evenings we would sit down to two meals that had both been spontaneously delivered. We did not know it was possible to feel so thoroughly loved and supported by an entire town. People stopped Rick daily to report they were praying for his wife. "How's your wife doing?" was a greeting he'd grown used to. I was on the prayer list at every single church in town. Two different churches organized meals to be delivered on a regular basis to our home. Astonishingly, we received well over a hundred meals during the year. People took care of our kids. Moms at the bus stop offered whenever or wherever to help with the kids – "Just let me know." Mom's talk about feeling like taxi drivers, but when the taxi is shut down, the logistics of four kids and their activities can get pretty intense. Our friends took care of it all. To know that every church prayed for me regularly is a thought that still sends tingles down my spine. Yes, we were supported by this small town, supported and carried through with awe-inspiring love. We felt absolutely overwhelmed with kindness and concern. We truly had never understood how many people cared about us, and we still stand in awe of people's goodness and concern.

Unbelievable encouragement, hope, and love poured out all over us; thank you, Lord!

Our treatment options were explained during the *tumor board*, a rather ominous gathering of white coats. We were definitely outnumbered by these men, who spewed odds and statistics as if we were in Vegas. I kept hearing "Five-year survival rate." This was craziness! Someone stop this bad movie, this can't be real. We were sitting in a small exam room, the white coats gathered 'round, each specialist accompanied by a couple mutts each.

"I want to live, and I want two breasts. What do I have to do?" I desperately wanted to look behind me, hoping to find someone else to whom they must be talking.

"Chemo first, eight rounds, followed by surgery and radiation."

One week later I was eye to eye with my first chemo nurse. "Tell me about your children. . ."

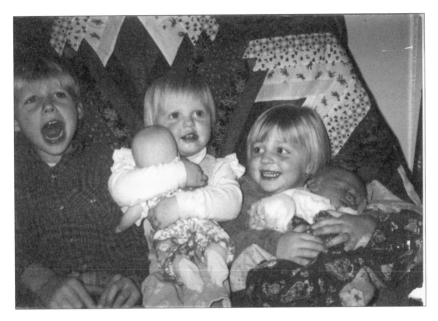

## 2

*Joel, Mallory, Kate, and baby Bryce at Christmas.*

# Incredibly Cute Kids

"I'm sorry, Honey, you'll need to wait thirty minutes before your next pain shot."

I was infuriated. I was in intense pain, and this placating nurse was trying to tell me, another nurse, that you had to wait *exactly* four hours between pain shots! It wasn't true! Somebody help me! Labor had been cruising along, a little pain, very uncomfortable, but doing the Lamaze huffing thing seemed to help. Rick had been at my side for twelve hours straight. "Go get something to eat, Honey, take a break, I'll be fine..." He had disappeared to the cafeteria when a thunderous contraction roared in. Calm, calm, four small breaths in, one long, one out...hee, hee, hee,

hee, whoo, hee, hee, hee, whoo. Yeah, right. It sounds good when you're lying on pillows with all the *pregos* practicing, but when the real pain hits, it's "Give me the shot!" The wave passed as Rick popped back in with a big smile on his face. I never resented him more. Look at him! He's in no pain at all! He gets one moment of pleasure; I get nine months of puking and discomfort, and now this...

"How are you doin', Hon?" I grabbed the collar of his shirt and pulled him down real close until I was sure he could hear me real well. Through gritted teeth I slowly growled, "Get the doctor and get me a pain shot . . . now!"

Eyes widened, he pulled back in shock. I think I got my point across. He took his tuna sandwich breath quickly out of the room. A few minutes later the worthless nurse reappeared with my syringe. "I understand you're in some pain, Honey?" Unfortunately, I discovered nothing really dulls the intense pain of childbirth. And nothing makes it disappear like catching the first glimpse of the beautiful miracle it produces. Joel Richard Howard was totally beautiful, he was perfect, and he became the joy of our lives.

When Joel was three months old, I reluctantly went back to work and Rick became Mr. Mom. With the car seat in the front of the truck, Joel went everywhere. When he was old enough to crawl around the back of the truck, it became his playpen. Rick would be up on a roof fixing something, and there was Joel, sucking on a pipe wrench in the back of the truck. Joel loved McDonald's, and Rick learned a hamburger could keep him occupied and quiet for long stretches of time. It became a daily stop. A donut for breakfast, hamburgers for lunch. My baby's nutrition was a disaster. His car seat acquired layers of chocolate sprinkles, catsup, mustard, and smeared hamburger buns. When the truck pulled into our yard in the afternoon, and I would run over to give my men a hug, I would find my beautiful baby covered in dried snot and catsup, filthy clothes... and a huge smile on his face.

How can we love another child like we love Joel? I seriously doubted I had enough love for another child, but I badly wanted to experience this miracle again. Kathleen Patricia solved the dilemma. Born two years later, this beautiful, smiling child quelled all doubts of enough love. Kate was calm, relaxed, smiling, and content. She was pure joy. While Joel roared around the house, Kate pushed contentedly around in her walker following *Doe Doe* wherever he went. I could sit her on a blanket, forget her, check on her an hour later, and she was still contentedly playing with the same pile of toys. And loving…this kid was a *snuggler.* She loved to bury her head in my neck. Her body would go totally limp, and she could lay there forever without moving. Total contentment.

When Kate came along, she stayed with a precious little Portuguese woman near my school so I could dash over during my lunch breaks to nurse and hold my little girl. At the end of the school year, I quit. I just wanted to be home with my babies.

Now Rick had two car seats in his truck. It was Joel's second home, and he didn't want to be left behind. Kate's first word was *Dahee! Dahee!* She loved going in the truck with dad. And mom loved the peace and quiet after they drove off!

I started quilting. We had spent October in New Hampshire visiting Rick's parents, George and MaryLu. His dad was a road construction manager, so they moved frequently to follow the jobs. We loved when they lived back East. It was a great area to visit, and they are gracious hosts. MaryLu is an amazing cook, and after a day of touring we would return to wonderful meals. She's one of those ladies who can disappear into the kitchen and a half hour later emerge with a mouth-watering meal. How does she do that?

Rick's memories of childhood start and end with his mom's great food. He woke up every morning to the smell of bread baking. She made a cake every day, and with five kids, they wiped up every bit of it. Rick's school lunches were the envy of every kid—sandwiches made of big slabs of homemade bread, a quarter of a cake. I can't even comprehend the volume of food he ate. MaryLu swears when Rick left home for college her grocery bill went down by $300.00 a month!

Obviously, opportunities to visit his mom and dad were a treat. Sometimes she would even keep the kids so Rick and I could go explore by ourselves. We loved the Amish country. Rick was enchanted with all the barns and farms. We spent days driving around looking for *Sale* signs. We pulled into the driveway, bought their apples or jam or whatever they had for sale. He didn't care; he just wanted a chance to talk to the Amish men about farming and their way of life. After a few minutes' conversation, we invariably were escorted on a tour of their farm as these gracious and gentle people hosted us. They were as fascinated with us as we were with them. At 6'7", Rick was clearly the tallest human they had seen. It was very entertaining to watch people greet him with incredulous stares.

The Amish can quilt—the quilts are absolutely beautiful. I wanted one badly. They were amazingly pricey, and after extensive shopping, I decided I would make my own. *Quilting in a Day* was a book that gave me a ray of hope. I didn't even like to sew, but if I could crank one out in a day. . .

Back at home, I attacked my project with gusto. It seemed to be pretty simple, lots of straight sewing and cutting. "I think I'll make a quilt for our bed!" A king-size quilt is not a recommended beginner project, but it worked for me. Time was something I had a lot of. With two little kids running around and a third on the way, I didn't get out much. I sewed with passion. Our friends were all having kids—a great excuse to make baby quilts. Birthday coming up? Wall hangings were a hit. Christmas? The quilting opportunities never ended. I was a maniac.

I quilted through the discomfort of my third pregnancy. Mallory Ann was a big blue-eyed, strawberry blonde beauty. And she let everyone know she had arrived. This kid was no cuddler. Mallory demanded action, and now! It felt like a tornado had hit. I quilted through the crying. I would tell myself to keep sewing as Mallory screamed in her crib before naptime. Mallory throwing another tantrum? I'd go sew a couple squares until she wore out. It was my salvation.

Every bed had a quilt—even the walls were covered. After I wore out my old machine, I moved on to the next. I could deal with three kids, as long as there were quilts to be made. We still wanted one more, though. Bryce Alan made four. This beautiful little boy made our family complete. He kicked and flopped like a whirling dervish for nine months and just kept on going once he got out. We had four kids in five years… and we were done!

Bryce loved to be *ouside*. Rick constructed a gate to tightly enclose our property so Bryce could roam. His daily uniform was rubber boots and a diaper. Anything else he took off. He entertained himself all day out there and cried when I brought him in for lunch. He would eat, pass out, and as soon as he woke up start yelling *"ouside."* I could toss him back out in the yard until dinner and together with Jake, our golden retriever, he explored the wilds.

We were standing in the kitchen. The kids had come in to inhale the cookies I had just pulled from the oven. We were gathered around the island. Rick wasn't home, but even if this wasn't exactly the right time, I just had to get it off my chest. "You know all those trips I've been taking this last week" Deep breath! "I've been going to Stanford for some tests." Their eyes widened, the chewing stopped. "I found out I have breast cancer." But I hurry on, "It's treatable, and they can get it out. It's just going to take some time and treatment."

"Are you going to be OK, Mom?"

"Yes, I'll be fine; it's just going to be a rough few months while they treat it." They asked a lot of questions about the treatment; mostly they wanted to know how it was going to affect their little lives. I portrayed my most confident and tough demeanor. They went back outside to play, and I went upstairs and cried.

I now regret all the emotion I hid from my kids. At the time, I thought I was protecting them. I now know it would have been healthier for all of us, if I had just let the kids see me cry. I think witnessing my emotions would have helped them process their own emotions. As it is, they still are reluctant to talk about how cancer really affected them. "*In due time…*"

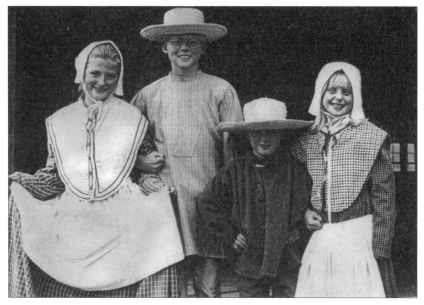

## 3

*The kids having fun with the Amish in Ohio.*

# Treatment Begins: Chemo One

I was scared, anxious, peaceful, trusting; each emotion surfaced and was then pulled down by the undercurrent. The riptide was strong. When peace surfaced, I turned my face upward and whispered Thanks.

How bad will it be? I had heard horror stories; I had also been encouraged to hear, "Ah, it's not that bad," this from a friend of a friend who had just finished treatment.

"Whatever it is, Lord, I can handle it…bring it on." Strolling confidently toward the Infusion Room, shoulders back, head held high, tightly gripping Rick's hand, I didn't speak. Nor did Rick. Checking in with an unenthusiastic employee in green scrubs, "Yes, Sandy Howard." I glance down; my name is in the appointment book. I realized I was still hanging on to the shred of hope that it really wasn't me that needed treatment. But no, there I am in *The Book*. "Sandy Howard." That's me. I have…deep sigh, cancer. I really do.

Mr. Enthusiasm points to a chair…be with you in a minute. Sitting, trying to act casual. What do you do before a massive dose of poison is injected into your body? Flip through a magazine, glance around the room at all the others? They're people with pink gasmask-looking devices sitting around the waiting room. Wow. That's unnerving. What's their story? What do they have? How do they feel? I try not to stare. Who in this room is going to live, who's going to die? I know I'm not gonna die, not this way anyhow. I attempt a smile and a nod to the lady across from me. She glances down. I have to go to the bathroom again, but I just did this . . . My hands are shaking as I pull the seat cover from the wall.

The Infusion Room, as it is officially called, was an ominous place. It contained people in varying stages of health. Some looked totally healthy and out of place. I would come to recognize them as first timers. The rest of us had that chemo look. We were in varying stages of baldness, dark circles under the eyes, a pasty complexion. The room had a slightly metallic, chemical odor to it that I came to despise. The greater room was partitioned off into four smaller cubicles; each cubicle was equipped with four chairs and a Barcalounger in the corner. Like being shown to your table in a restaurant, we were met by a nurse who led us to our spot for the day.

It's my turn. Mr. Enthusiasm leads. I go first, Rick follows. "I wonder if he appreciates his health." *Compromised Patient Area* above my head. I am *not* compromised. I am healthy. I will not allow my body to be compromised. And then the smell. I hate the smell of chemicals, so unhealthy. The irony assaults me.

My little cubicle has three chairs and a bed. "What the heck," I think, as I flop on the bed. Warmed blankets are placed over me. Nurses are such wonderful people.

The total process amazingly takes several hours, most of it spent waiting. Once the IV is started, the fluid takes several hours to slowly infuse. After I tell Mary about my kids, I settle back on the bed and the tears slowly leak out. "I will not cry through this process," I vow. "Suck it up, be tough." It was a mentality I had established early in life.

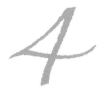

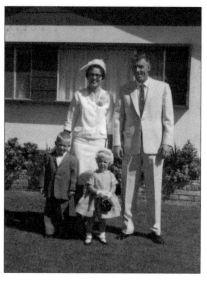

*My mom and dad, Dave and me on Easter Sunday.*

# T-town and More

I was raised in the small town of Turlock, California, in a wonderful middle class family. My parents were both hard working. My dad was a truck driver, and I had the distinct advantage of having a mom who, rather than work, chose to stay home with my brother, Dave, and me. My earliest memory is lying on my mom's big, puffy bed, rolling around giggling as she tickled me. I knew I was thoroughly loved. My mom was my best buddy. We did everything together. As long as I can remember, I had my hand in her back pocket wherever we walked. That was just how I did it. My dad called her Hon, and that was what Dave and I called her too. When he was in the eighth grade, he decided calling your mom "Hon" wasn't cool and went through a painful period of trying to break the habit. He finally gave in. She's been Hon to us all ever since.

Hon is an amazing lady. She is one of those rare persons able to break the cycle of abuse. My grandmother was, OK, I'll just say it, mean! She had a knack for making everyone around her miserable. Hon's job from the time she was twelve was to get up at 4:30 a.m. and fix breakfast for her brother and dad before they went out to work on the ranch at 6:00 a.m. She had to start dinner every day when she got home from school. She still remembers the brutal punishment when her mom arrived home one day and the potatoes weren't peeled. She was also the housekeeper for as far back as she can remember. In her spare time, she provided manual labor in the almond orchard my grandpa farmed.

She gratefully married my dad at eighteen and got the heck out of there. But frequent migraine headaches remain an unrelenting reminder of her unhappy childhood. She vividly recalls her first migraine in the fourth grade, and I vividly recall her dark bedroom when the dreaded migraine would hit. "I just need to sleep, Honey, I'll be better tomorrow," to the sound of her feet frantically pounding as she dashed to the bathroom to be sick. I would have done anything to make her feel better. I felt so helpless and frustrated knowing she was suffering behind that closed door. I went out of my way to ensure I never upset her, fearing it might trigger a migraine. There were heating pads, stinky muscle relaxant rubs, ice packs, and drives to the chiropractor with Hon hunched and stiff behind the wheel. Turning her head at all caused the sickening pain that could induce another round of vomiting, so I would be her eyes and ears as she slowly guided the giant black *Batmobile* Cadillac to the chiropractor's office for "an adjustment." She tried all the latest and greatest drugs as they came out, all to no avail.

But the one sure trigger for a migraine was a visit to grandma's house. I resented my grandmother for continuing to cause my mom pain. Vague memories of my grandmother range from fear, to disgust, to repulsion. "Give grandma a hug," mercifully stopped early in elementary school. Her smell was very unpleasant; her chin whiskers rubbed my face. By third grade, I was allowed to stay outside during the obligatory visits to their ranch. I would walk around in the huge greasy-smelling shop my brother found so fascinating, hoping we could leave soon.

The only thing my grandmother gave me was a small china doll. She called me into the house and handed me the doll. I looked at my first gift curiously thinking, "Why did she give me this ugly doll?" I knew I needed to be polite and act as if I liked it, but I couldn't fathom this sudden kindness. She had missed all my birthdays; they just didn't give gifts. Now she told me the doll was very valuable, and I needed to take good care of it. My heart filled with dread as I realized this gift warranted a thank-you kiss. It took some time to summon the courage. I took a deep breath and stood on my tiptoes to kiss grandma on the cheek. I could sense her stiff, unyielding body as I lightly balanced myself with a touch on her arm. She stared straight ahead and gruffly reminded me to "Take good care of it."

Out in the shop I followed Dave around as he explored all the greasy tools. I held the doll by her dress, anxious to dump this thing in the car and be done with it. When Hon finally called for us to go, I breathed a sigh of relief and hurried toward the car. Incredibly, along the way, I tripped over a metal bar. My heart stopped as I watched that china head shatter against the cement floor. I stood frozen, horrified. Dave ran to get Hon, who hurried over to scoop me up in consolation. "I'm so sorry, Honey. It was just an accident. She shouldn't have given that to you; you're too young for something like that." I was never so glad to leave Grandma's house.

By high school, I wasn't required to go to their house, and their visits to our home were confined to Thanksgiving and Christmas. My grandfather rarely spoke, and when he did, he was gruff. Twice a year was plenty for me. My grandmother died when I was eighteen. I was appalled at the excitement I felt when I learned Grandma had been admitted to the hospital, gravely ill. I experienced a huge sense of relief when I learned she had died. She would finally stop tormenting my precious mom. No one shed a tear at the funeral.

Thankfully, my dad came from a wonderful, healthy household. His father died before I was born, but Frank Knapp was a model father and husband. Martha Knapp was my real grandma. A tall, thin Swedish woman, she was well known and loved in our community. Grandma was a devout Christian woman, a pillar of faith and love. When I was growing up, she lived in "the house in the alley," a cozy bungalow I loved to visit. She only lived a few blocks away, so I loved to walk to Grandma's house. One thing you could count on, Grandma would be baking. A wonderful smell always wafted from her kitchen. She relentlessly cranked out muffins, breads, and cookies to deliver to friends and relatives. Grandma liked to make muffins in those little mini pans, you know, the ones that make muffins a perfect mouthful. I downed many mouthfuls during visits. I ate zucchini muffins before I learned there was actually a vegetable in there and carrot muffins even after I learned she had sneaked a nasty veggie in. I loved to plop down at her little table for two and anticipate her delicious treats. The muffins or cookies were always served with a small cup of juice. She was a master at Riis Scrun Scrit, a Swedish rice pudding that was her trademark dish. Nobody made it like grandma. The rice was always perfectly soft, fluffy, and slightly sweet and sprinkled with cinnamon sugar and topped with milk. It was mouthwatering.

When I spent the night, I got to sleep in her bed. She was so soft and warm and always smelled so good. I loved snuggling with her. In the morning, she always made Swedish pancakes. Huge, paper-thin pancakes with jam and powdered sugar all rolled into a thin log. I could power them down faster than she could make them. A closet in her living room contained toys for the grandkids, and she had a pretty little backyard to play with them.

If someone was sick, you could count on Grandma's big blue bomber gliding up to the front of the house. She just always knew. If we had a cold or flu, it was chicken noodle soup. Sprained ankle, big test coming up? She delivered muffins or a bowl of Riis Scrun Scrit. "I just made up a batch in the double boiler, Honey," she would encourage, with her soothing voice. "You eat this; it will make you feel better."

Grandma was a foot rubber. Each of her four sons, thirteen grandkids, and thirty-four great grandkids could tell you a story about grandma rubbing their feet. I remember lying on the couch with my feet in Grandma's soft lap. She was fond of *tsk'ing*—you know that sound that's made when you put the tip of your tongue against the back of your front teeth. "Tsk, tsk, tsk, now, Honey, you have to learn to take care of yourself." Any admonition was welcomed, as long as she kept rubbing.

She was also a big fan of Vicks, that obnoxious smelling Mentholatum rub. After the steaming, inviting chicken soup, you could count on a good slather. "Just rub your chest real good with this." After a while, we learned to just lay still. It didn't matter how much we squirmed, we were going to be slathered anyway. An old rag and two safety pins nailed the job down. But she wasn't done yet. "Hot compresses will break up that nasty cough, Honey. Now just lay still." Her treatments ended with a heartfelt prayer for our health and healing, "In *Jesus*' name!" She was my real grandma, a matriarch in the truest sense, and I love her dearly.

I loved kids; I loved babysitting. I just plain loved people. I loved school, all the action, and the opportunity for sports. We didn't have recreation teams for kids back then, so I couldn't wait to get to junior high and play on a team. I had talked my dad into installing a hoop in the driveway and spent many hours practicing my jump shot. I begged for a pitch back for Christmas, one of those nets you throw at, and the ball bounces back. I spent hours being Vida Blue in the backyard. I had a mean fastball and a gap between my front teeth that allowed me to spit just like Reggie Jackson. I listened to every Oakland A's game on my little AM radio and daily clipped game articles from the newspaper for my scrapbook. I was a major fan, and a serious tomboy.

Finally, in the sixth grade, I could be on a team. I loved basketball. I loved competition. The volleyball team was fun, but that was just to keep me occupied until basketball season started. After basketball came track or softball. I picked track because my friends were on the team, and I became fairly proficient at the high jump. I loved being outside; I loved working out. The high jump I could take or leave; it just allowed me to be part of the team.

It was during high school that I discovered a love for the sciences. I dreamed of being a pediatrician and driving around in a beat up Volkswagen van. I wasn't particularly fond of VWs—it was more of a disguise thing. I figured I was going to be successful at whatever I did, but I didn't want to brag about all the money I was going to make. I figured that if I drove around in an old VW, no one would guess how successful I was.

My favorite class was German, because the instructor was so cute and fun. Frau Rektor was bubbly and full of energy. She made learning a foreign language fun. She had connections in Switzerland, and I was one of the fortunate, chosen few to experience a summer working in Switzerland. I remember standing in the kitchen pleading with my dad to allow me to go. "I promise I'll pay you back with the money I make during the summer!" He was adamantly opposed to the idea of his daughter flying to Europe with a few other high-school kids, but with my mom petitioning steadily on my behalf, we prevailed.

I loved being on my own. I rented a room at a pensione but was disappointed to find my roommate a snotty rich girl from Los Angeles.

Veronica had a boyfriend back home and really did not want to be there. She was a source of fascination to me, as she had no appreciation for what I felt was the experience of a lifetime. We both worked at Migros, a large grocery store chain, but I rarely associated with her. She had such a negative attitude. I didn't want people associating me with her, so I kept my distance. She was my first spoiled brat experience, which only reinforced my VW van theory. If this is what money produced, I didn't want any part of it.

Migros had a fruit and vegetable stand out in front of the store. After a couple of days stuck stocking shelves, they thankfully moved me out front where the California girl could "razzle dazzle." Swiss German is a different dialect from High German, the language I learned in school. When I got off the plane in Zurich, I seriously thought I was in the wrong country. People were jabbering Swiss, and I could only make out a few words. I experienced a moment of panic before adjusting to the rhythm of their beautiful language.

Now I got to be outside, working at the fruit stand, and I loved it! People were so kind and receptive to the Californian. I had long blonde hair and was amazed to learn most Europeans thought everyone in California had blonde hair and lived in Hollywood. I only reinforced their stereotype. They were very gracious with me as I learned their language. As the summer wore on, I became comfortable with the Swiss dialect. Weekends were spent wandering the city, taking train excursions around their gorgeous country, and generally squeezing in as much fun as I could.

When our contract was complete, we had two glorious weeks to travel Europe. I bought a Eurail pass, and along with Kym, a fellow Turlock High student who had worked at a neighboring village, explored Italy, Germany, and Austria. Dad was right; I spent all my money over there and never did pay him back.

I dreamed of playing college ball. Women's scholarships were pretty rare, but it was my dream. Could I make it at the college level? Dad had other plans. "It's time to work and start earning your own way." Unfortunately there is a college located conveniently in Turlock, affectionately known as Turkey Tech. It was close, inexpensive, and I could live at home. It was everything I didn't want in a college. I enviously watched other friends go out of town to major universities; but, oh well, an education is an education. I loaded up on math and sciences, confidently declared pre-med, and was stunned at the level of difficulty of these classes. As a straight-A student in high school, I had never worked very hard for my grades. Suddenly I was working very hard for my Bs and Cs. After the first year, my guidance counselor recommended I change my major. It was a major blow for me. I just knew I would be a pediatrician. I didn't have a back-up plan. There was nothing else I wanted to do. I blindly took this man's advice, a decision I still regret.

I stuck with the sciences and applied to the nursing school at Fresno State. When I retook a couple of classes to get into the nursing program, I discovered just how important teachers could be. The same classes I got Cs in, I now got As in. Oh well, I was on a new path and I enjoyed nursing school. It was a good fit. When I got to the pediatrics rotation, I knew I had found my love. Kids are so fun. They are not hypochondriacs, they don't whine, they just get better as fast as they can and go home.

I had just accepted a job at Valley Children's Hospital when Rick and I decided to get married. There was no way I was moving to Los Banos. It was smaller than the hick town in which I had grown up. No, thank you. I asked him if he would consider moving to Fresno. His rental business was booming, he worked long hours, and he toyed with the idea of actually moving to Fresno. I felt so relieved. It didn't take long to see that his moving wasn't at all practical—and I was happy to do whatever it took to be with this wonderful man.

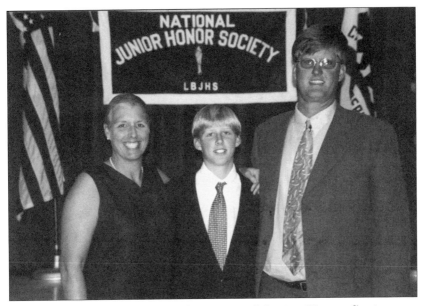

*Rick, Joel and me at Joel's National Junior Honor Society award banquet.*

# Hair Loss Extravaganza

I received my treatments every three weeks, and always on Tuesdays. Theoretically I was supposed to feel better by the weekend, and, usually by Monday, I was feeling well enough to go to work. I really enjoyed my job and wanted to continue to lead as normal a life as possible for as long as possible. I heard about the cumulative effects of chemo, but I left that in God's hands.

When all the fluid was pushed in, I felt tingly, slightly nauseated, repulsed at what had just occurred. I asked to use the restroom before the next tube was injected. Pushing my IV pole down the hall, I thought about how surreal this whole experience was. As a hospital RN, I had watched many people push their IV poles around in my time. I had always wondered what it must feel like to be "sick," to walk around attached to the pole. I struggled to maneuver the IV around the restroom—I was shocked and sickened when I saw the bright red water in the toilet bowl. "Dear God, my body has totally assimilated this poison. It's completely in my system now."

I couldn't embrace the concept of this agent helping me; I felt so healthy. There had not been one indicator of any illness. Yet, here I was. I felt like I was letting them poison a temple of God. I felt guilty. As my beautiful husband Rick drove me home from our first treatment, I was surprised at how good I felt. "I can do this, I can do this, only seven treatments left, only seven treatments left. Is this really happening? Is this a nightmare I'll wake up from?"

Anti-nausea meds are powerful. I was armed with three different kinds, and they worked. A baby pill, a mama pill, and the daddy pill, which was used every four hours for the first three days. After that, the serious nausea took a rest. Mama pill for the next couple of days, and the baby pill finished out the week until I felt pretty good. "This isn't so bad!" I thought after the first week.

I had been given lots of advice about the hair loss thing. "As soon as it starts to fall out, just shave it. It's the easiest way to handle it." All right, just shave it. But the thought of *just shaving it* consistently gave me chills, major shivers down my spine. Just shave it. I had prayed that this particular side effect would pass me by. Like the Angel at Passover, I mentally put a mark over my head. There, Lord, I can deal with a lot, but I really don't want to deal with this part. If you could just pass over me with this bald thing, I would really appreciate it. I sent out prayer requests on the prayer chain, "Baldness approaching. Please pray that Sandy does not go bald."

I work as a school nurse Monday through Wednesday. On the following Tuesday morning, as I brushed my hair for work, clumps of hair stuck in my brush. The tingling started again in my stomach. "Oh God, you're going to allow me to go bald." And I had so vigorously prayed that this side effect would pass me by. "OK, Lord, here's the deal. Please let the hair stay on my head until Wednesday, then I'll have four days to adjust to baldness before I have to go to work and face everybody on Monday."

I normally swim during my lunch break in the big, beautiful Merced College pool. This activity was suspended for a couple of days to save wear and tear on my hair. No washing, minimal brushing, I felt like it was ready to slide off my head. My scalp was tingly, a constant reminder of what was to come. After work on Wednesday, I went directly upstairs to brush my hair. This was it. Either God was going to directly intervene right now, or the hair was coming off. Dear God, clumps, clumps, and more clumps. It was definitely coming out. I was panicked. I flopped on my bed and cried. "I'm going to look like a freak. Lord, I really don't want to do this!" I got up and looked at my pillow covered with my hair. It was sickening. I walked back in the bathroom and looked in the mirror; there was a trail of hair on the floor behind me. "All right, Howard, suck it up. This is going to happen, and you're not going to make a big deal of it."

My girls were home from school. "Mallory, Kate, can you come in the garage?"

"Are you OK, Mom?"

"It's time to shave my head."

The girls had a sullen, repulsed look. "Are you serious, Mom?"

"I can gag on it at night on my pillow, or we can just buzz it off right now." I sat down by the workbench, pulled out the clippers that had served me well over the years, and held them up.

"I can't do it, Mom," said Kate.

"I'll do it. Give them to me." Mallory grabbed the clippers from my hand.

"Don't cry, don't cry," I kept telling myself as Mallory made slow and steady paths over my head. "I want to save the hair, maybe we can make hair to hang out from a hat." A friend had related how they had created a strip of hair that was velcroed to a baseball hat. I wanted at least to try to keep some of my own hair on my head, in any way possible. It was worth a try. After a quick glance in the mirror, "Don't think, don't think, and just keep moving." It was a blotchy butch, definitely in need of a hat. I pulled my cap on and rushed to the car. "Time to pick up Joel from soccer. I'll be right back." I allowed myself to cry all the way to the junior high school. "That's enough; now suck it up, Howard."

Joel jumped in the car, "Wow, Mom!"

"Yeah, I've got a new do!"

"Wow, Mom."

"Yeah, Buddy, it's going to be a long journey."

Hair was everywhere. It was so gross. The sewing machine was set up in the dining room. The ironing board was set up in the kitchen. The box of hair was on the kitchen counter. I shuttered as I looked around. Dana is super clean, and I knew it had to be grossing her out too. "Don't' worry about it. I'll just vacuum it up when we're done," she casually waved her hand. "No problem."

I don't know, I'm one of those people who get grossed out by a hair in the bathroom sink. Here was my hair all over her kitchen. You know how when a full cup gets bumped and water sloshes over the edge . . . I felt like I was ready to slosh. Tears welled up, "Don't cry, don't cry, just hang on 'till you get home."

Dana had a vision. None of us knew what we were doing, but she was on a mission. She took some of that wonder-under, the sticky stuff you use to mend holes in the kids' jeans and cut a long strip that measured ear to ear. When laid flat, hair that had been uniformly trimmed was placed along the strip. Another equal-sized piece of sticky stuff was laid on top to form a hair sandwich—that's a sick thought—and lots of ironing and sewing later, a strip of hair was created. This strip was attached to the inside of a baseball cap with Velcro, and if you didn't look too close, it looked like I had thin hair hanging out from under my hat. This sounds simple, but it was quite a project. Much of the hair I saved was all wadded up and difficult to use. We ended up digging around in the box, scrounging for enough long pieces. "Here's a chunk that's long enough!" Sweeping pieces off the counter, "This chunk will fill in that space." A couple friends stopped by, a bottle of wine was opened. A couple more friends stopped by. It was a party.

My sister-in-law appeared. Pam is an amazingly gifted artist and photographer. She handed me a photo album and said, "You'd better sit down." I opened a treasure: She had compiled pictures of family and friends. Adjacent to each picture was a scripture verse or inspirational quote. "It's to inspire you during your chemo treatments." I was stunned and touched. This was such a beautiful and loving gift. I couldn't imagine how much time she had taken to compose this beautiful treasure.

"Oh, yes, that one is just perfect! Wonderful color, yes, definitely. I like this one!" exclaimed the overly enthusiastic sales clerk. The tones are just perfect! I glanced cautiously at Dana, giving her a what-do-you-think look. She gave a slight side-to-side wag. "I guess it's OK. Yeah, I like it." She was definitely on the spot. I found myself unwilling and physically unable to look in the mirror. The little swirly barber chair was swirled dead to the left. "Here!" wig mama enthused, "let's just take a little off the bangs, and it will be just right!" It was all up to Dana.

"If you like this one, then let's get out of here. Yeah, we can take it to Eddie. If it needs any trimming he can fix it up, and I bet it'll look great." I looked around the shop—skin cream for cancer patients: "Chemotherapy dries out your skin! Our lotion will protect you from the ravaging effects" proclaimed a sign in the corner. Wow, lotions, shampoos, makeup, all proclaiming to soften the effects of chemo. Someone is making a lot of money off people like me, I thought uncomfortably. We are definitely a captive and desperate audience. "Let's just take it to Eddie, my hairstylist" Dana did not look happy or confident. "Now, remember, once it's trimmed, you can't bring it back," wig mama chirped as she snipped a couple hairs off the bangs.

"Yeah, whatever," I thought. "Just let me out of here." My throat was tight, and I felt sick as I handed Dana the keys and headed for the door. I needed some quiet. There was so much going on in my head that I felt one more ounce of input would tip me over the edge into a scary place I didn't want to go. I found a little patch of grass in the hot parking lot under an aspiring tree and let it out. It felt so good to cry. My cup was full, and crying put me back down to seven-eights cup. "All right, Howard, that's enough, suck it up." I was sniffling and wiping as Dana came out with an ominous looking bag. We sat in her van with the AC blasting as I flipped to I Peter. This had become my favorite chapter in the last couple of weeks, especially 5:9 "Humble yourself before God, and in due time He will exalt you because He loves and cares for you."

"Can you read the whole chapter to me?" I felt calm and peace as Dana read the reassuring words. "All right, thanks; better get over to Eddie and see what he can do."

"Oh my gosh! This is awful!" Eddie had pulled the wig onto my head. I looked in the mirror and shuddered. Eddie gushed on, "Who sold you this wig? Oh, it's terrible! The tones are all wrong!" I cringed as I thought he might hit me in his rage and despair. This was clearly the worst thing that had happened to him today. And, of course, the entire shop had turned to view the horror he was proclaiming. Dana mouthed c a n c e r and pointed to me so people would stop staring at the spectacle.

"You get her on the phone right now and tell her you want to take this wig back!" Well, OK, I thought. Wig mama and I had a short conversation, "I cut it. I can't take it back!"

Her proclamation sounded final. I put the phone on my chest and looked at Eddie pleadingly, "She says she won't take it back because she already cut it." "She what? Give me that phone. This wig is awful! You have to take it back!" Silence. "Then you're going to hear from my lawyer!" I'm not much for threatening people, or lawyers for that matter, but at that moment it sounded pretty good to me. Yeah, Eddie, go! But now what? "You call your bank right now and have them stop that check." All right, sounded good to me. One call later, I was holding an unpaid-for wig and desperate to get this shopping trip over with. There are two other places in Fresno that sell wigs. Eddie gave us directions as we hustled out the door.

Back in Dana's van, we blasted to wig store number one, where a line of mini cheerleaders were queued up to buy their prosthetic pony-tails. Now there's a concept. The sales person gave us a "Get-in-line-and-wait-your-turn-Buddy" look. Thankfully, the second wig place was a to-tal blessing. We walked in and breathed a sigh of relief. Let me just say, a wig store is overwhelming. I stood in the middle of the shop and gave it a 360. Oh my gosh! Wigs hanging on the walls like hunting trophies, wigs stacked on the counters, wigs everywhere. I felt my cup fill back up. I vowed not to cry.

I've never been very good with hair; in fact, it was usually just in my way. That was until a few days ago when it came out. Now I just wanted my own hair back. Friends had suggested I take this opportunity to *experiment*. "Heck, get a redheaded curly wig!"

"Yeah, great idea." I would smile weakly, trying not to cry. I had never been excited about my own hair, yet now I searched for an exact replica. I just wanted to look like me. No stares, ogles, or questions. I just wanted to fade into the crowd.

Dana explained our situation to the sympathetic saleswoman. "Let me see, sweetheart, we'll find you just the right hairpiece." I grabbed one that reminded me of Meg Ryan in her last movie. "I like this one. . ." I started feeling positive . . . maybe I could spark up my image. Twenty minutes later, it was over. This wig cost one-half the price the cancer store charged and came with a guarantee. It had been a long day. I would come home to a phone message from wig mama making massive apolo-gies. I mailed her wig back the next day. I had a new do.

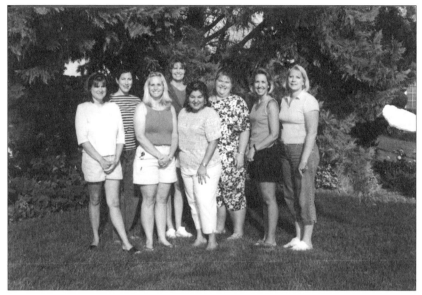

*Our bible study group.*

# The Toilet . . . I Mean The Baths

It was an amazing group of ladies God had assembled. I had felt led to invite our neighborhood ladies to a Bible study. Ann was the only one to show up the first week, but soon the living room was full. They really were an exceptional group. I thought I was reaching out to them. In the end, I clearly saw how God used this group to reach out and support me through my treatment.

I was curled in my usual spot on one end of our cozy couch. I had just shared my news with the group. Monica came over and hugged me. As she held me, she whispered in my ear, "You are such an awesome person. We know you are going to make it through this. If there's anything we can do at any time, we will be here for you." You know how you're never sure what to say to someone who is in crisis? Say that. We prayed and cried together. I drew great strength from them.

God works in amazing ways . . . like how I ended up in Los Banos. And no, it does not mean *the toilet*; it means "the baths." You see, the padres used to walk over the hills from their missions on the coast looking for more converts. Along the way, they discovered these natural pools of water in beautiful rock formations. The padres stopped to soak and relax in these pools, and they became known as "The Baths" or Los Banos. When I caught my first glimpse of the beautiful baths, the Silicon Valley had yet to be born. Los Banos was a sleepy little town where everyone knew everyone. You left your home unlocked and left the keys in your truck. Rick was well known in his town—local boy made good. He had attended UOP on a football scholarship, was an up and coming entrepreneur, and at twenty-eight was a young school board member. Our first date in Los Banos was a dinner-dance, fundraiser event. I met at least 300 people that night. Most were very gracious. Some were very curious about who Rick Howard would be dating. I did feel somewhat awkward being on display that night, yet proud to be with this obviously respected man.

Rick truly is and was a unique individual. Although he already owned several homes that he rented out, he chose to live in "The Condo," a metal shop located on a piece of property in the country with two rental homes. When his parents moved to New Mexico he needed a free place to sleep, and, yes, he is a major tightwad . . . so he renovated the little office in the front corner of his shop, moved in a bed, and named it The Condo. The condo was spartan living at its best. A small bedroom, small bathroom, living room, and "kitchen," which was actually a dent in the wall with a sink. There was no fridge, no food; he ate what he could get for free. One time when his brother was hauling corn nuts, Rick ended up with a few cases. He ate them for lunch for months. When he got hungry for dinner, he would pop in at his friends' house, a different one each night.

Our first dinner/date at the condo was a classic. He had arranged an old couch in front of the little fireplace in the main shop area. We were quaintly surrounded by pipe parts, spare doors, windows, and lumber. As he escorted me to his "formal living area," he opened a box of Triscuits and poured them onto a paper plate. "Hors de oeuvres are served." There was an inviting fire crackling in the little stove in which he had constructed a swinging grill. He flopped a couple of huge steaks on the grill, swung it back over the fire, and cooked dinner. A couple of foil-wrapped potatoes were pulled from the bottom of the fire, and our meal was complete. I was impressed.

When we married, the condo was our logical first home since we could live there for free. We opted to save all of my paychecks from Los Banos Hospital, where I had taken a job, so we could buy more property. Our first mutual purchase was H Street—a two-acre parcel with ten houses. This place was badly run down and required a lot of work. Rick tore into it like a tornado. Within a couple of months, all the houses were fixed and rented out. He even converted a garage on the property to another living unit. We had a positive cash flow.

Since he was on the school board, he was invited to attend school board conventions for free. Free room, free food. Oh yes, this was a good thing. One of our first trips was to one of the nicer hotels in San Francisco. We cruised up in Rick's old work truck and pulled into line at the Saint Francis Hotel. The bellman came up to the truck and casually asked Rick if he knew he was in line for the Saint Francis. "Yeah, I know."

"Can I see your reservations, please, sir?"

"Sure. No problem." This was my VW van dream come true. This guy thought we were a couple of vagrants.

"I'm sorry, sir; we'll be right with you . . ." I didn't own luggage, so I had filled an old duffle bag with my stuff. We looked good as we unloaded his truck.

We had an amazing weekend. The party on the first night was a reception at the top of the Saint Francis, hosted by an architectural firm anxious to build one of our new schools. There were huge prawn platters, every kind of cold cut, fancy like neither one of us had ever seen. I had worn my dressiest pair of slacks, which was actually one step up from jeans, but I felt like I had outdone myself. Rick, thankfully, owned one sport jacket. We were looking good. Or so we thought, as we tried to gain entrance to the party.

"Excuse me, sir, this is a private party." We were abruptly stopped at the door by the tuxedoed man.

"We have tickets."

"May I see them, please?" Heads turned as we walked in. Who let their children come? was the standard look of disapproval and surprise.

This was the fifty- to seventy-year-old crowd in their evening gowns and tuxedoes! We were definitely out of place. Time for a plan: We decided to eat and drink as much as possible, as quickly as possible, so we could go have some fun.

"I'll go and get the beer; you go and pile as many of those prawns as you can on a plate, and we'll meet back here." I swiftly strode over to the bar (a jog would have definitely been tacky), and asked the bartender what kind of beer they had.

"Beer?" I matched his incredulous look.

"Yes, beer."

"We'll have to call downstairs to get some delivered, Ma'am." Unbelievable. What were these old folks drinking, anyway? Mr. Tuxedo disgustedly handed over two Coors Lights. Back at our spot, Rick had already devoured half of the plate of prawns. We hunkered over the plate, eating and drinking as fast as we could. Unfortunately, I had ingested a large mouthful of liquid when one of our fellow misfits, an older man in a cowboy getup, cracked a joke. I choked, and to my horror, spewed my mouthful of suds on the Persian rug. I glanced around, hoping no one had seen, and knew it was time to scram. We opted for a take-out meal. And with a couple of cold-cut sandwiches and beers stuffed in our pockets, we went in search of the cable cars.

Our next vacation was a trip to San Diego. We actually bought airline tickets, a huge splurge for us. Of course, it was the annual school board convention, so our room was paid for. Los Banos was still looking to build new schools, and architects were swarming. Every night a different firm took us out to dinner. We were living large at the fanciest restaurants. One night I was shocked to have a plate of sixty-dollar abalone placed in front of me. I didn't know food could cost that much. I had recently taken a job in Dos Palos as their school nurse. I figured I'd just call in sick a couple of days and make it a nice, long weekend. My superintendent, Dr. Big, would also be attending the conference, but odds were I would never see him. They would never know I played hooky.

Rick strolled into the beautiful, spacious lobby to check in while I pulled luggage from the little rental car. There was Dr. Big. "He's staying in our hotel!"

"No way!" Hmmm, gonna have to be careful. Not only was he in our hotel, but his room was on our floor. Hmmm, could be trouble . . . The next morning I gracefully dove behind the bushes as Dr. Big strolled

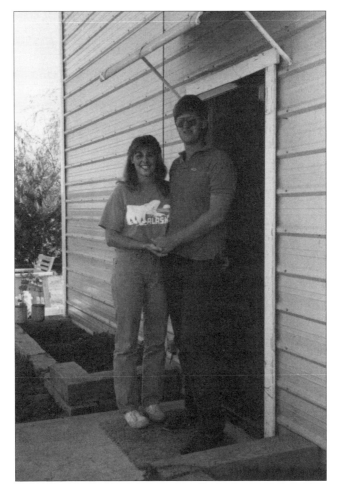

*The newlyweds proudly pose in front of "The Condo."*

by. We had to run surveillance each time we left or returned to our room. I felt like James Bond. I saw more of Dr Big that weekend than I ever had at work, and, no, he never did see me.

Back at the condo, things had been spruced up. The shop had no windows, so I found an oversized screen in the shop and tacked it to the open front door. Fresh air! A breeze filtered through. I was in heaven. When Rick came home, he was struck with a great idea. "You know what, Hon? I could install a screen door!"

"Could you really?" He disappeared into the shop. Rick watched newspaper ads for auctions and liquidation sales and always had spare parts for the growing number of rentals. Our shop was also the dumping ground for anybody doing a remodel job. People dropped off light fixtures, toilets, sinks. We had it all handily stored in our "formal" living room. He leafed through the screen doors as if through a rack of pants until he found the perfect fit. Fifteen minutes later, it was a done deal. I was a happy wife.

We had a small, black and white TV with rabbit ears, which you had to be very motivated to watch to endure the fuzz. We didn't watch much TV. Our radio was a small AM job, so forget the music. Our entertainment was sitting outside on our little patch of Bermuda grass watching the renters.

Kurtis and Debbie lived in an 800-square-foot house about forty yards from our new screen door. She was a screamer. I felt sorry for her kids. One evening we were reclining in our lawn chairs on our freshly mowed patch, enjoying the cool evening. We watched as a tow truck slowly eased down the driveway. We exchanged a curious look and settled in. The driver backed up to Debbie's beat-up little truck and methodically began to attach chains. We smiled and nodded at each other. This was going to be good. It didn't take long for Debbie to come flying out the front door in full rage. "What the H...do you think you're doing?" Her arms were swinging wildly; her whole body was bent forward. Unfortunately we couldn't hear their conversation, but we were able to distinguish a few expletives. After their chat, the man calmly went back to hitching up the little truck. Debbie was small, but she was ferocious. She was not slowing down. The longer he worked, the louder she screamed.

"Can I get you something to drink, Hon?"

"No, no, sit back down. I don't want you to miss any of this." Mission completed. Tow-truck man climbed in his truck seemingly unfazed by Debbie's continuing tirade. As he slowly pulled away, Debbie reached into the back of his truck and yanked out a tire iron. "When can I get my truck back, you M---F---er? Give me a time and a date, you M----F----er!" In a final act of desperation, she swung her little arm back, discus style, and heaved the tire iron at the back of the tow truck, shattering his back window. Tow-truck man didn't speed up, nor did he slow down. He didn't even duck. He just rumbled slowly out of the driveway. We were transfixed as we watched the back of the little truck bump away.

We were caught off guard seeing Debbie strolling our way. "Uh, Rick, could I use your phone for a minute please?" she purred in the sweetest drawl.

"Sure, Debbie." We eavesdropped unashamedly as Debbie related the event to Kurtis.

"Uh, Honey, a man just repossessed our truck. . . Yeah, he just drove off with it. He wouldn't tell me when I could get it back . . . yeah . . . oh, and there was a little problem," she drawled on. "Yeah, I sorta broke his window . . . yeah, I did, but I didn't mean to. . . OK, Honey, bye."

I finally realized my mouth was hanging open. I made a solid attempt to shut it and appear unfazed as she hung up the phone. "Thanks, Rick.

"Yeah, you're welcome, Debbie. Have a nice evening. . ."

There was a nasty flu going around that winter, and I was sick as a dog. I had been in bed two days moaning, only leaving to crawl to the bathroom to puke. By day three, I perked up enough to trudge the three steps it took to get to the couch. I sat there in my bathrobe with my long hair matted and greasy, just thankful to be alive. By noon, I had the strength to walk the two more steps required to get to the "kitchen." Although we now had a refrigerator, it was a wasted effort. The fridge was empty. I slumped back to the couch to contemplate my options. I could shower and drive to town . . . Not! I could wait for Rick to get home from working and hope he brought food, or I could brave *The Rooster*.

Rick was raised in the country and had this thing for animals. If there was a patch of grass, he fenced it and put some sheep or goats in to mow it. Free feed. Whatever. We had goats in the little pasture to the right—a whole different story to be told—and sheep in the big pasture to the left. Tucked behind the shop was the chicken pen. People rave about fresh farm eggs. I even know people who make special trips to get their eggs fresh. I truly couldn't tell the difference. An egg was an egg. And I knew there were eggs just beyond the metal wall that I was sitting in front of. The only thing between me and that egg, though, was *The Rooster*. This cocky fella didn't bother anyone but me. My two-year nephew could waltz right in the pen, gather eggs, and stroll back out. Rick? Not a problem. Me? I would get within twenty feet of the coop, and he would cock his ugly little head back, raising his wings up. If he could hiss, he would have. Naturally, I let Rick gather the eggs. But in desperate times, I would arm myself with a shovel and, swinging, grab as many eggs as I could before slamming the rickety door behind me.

These were desperate times. On my way through the shop I grabbed a shovel and determinedly walked into the coop. "Come on, you ugly little runt," I growled at my friend as he cocked his little head back and menacingly raised his wings. The fight was on. He dodged a couple of swings, and while he was off balance, I grabbed a couple of eggs. Feeling pretty smug, I popped out of the coop and looked up to find a Sheriff standing in my path. "Uh, hello, can I help you?"

He gave me a curious, concerned look. "There have been some thefts reported out in this area. I was just driving through, thought I'd check on any suspicious people."

"Oh, OK." *Just get out of my way, Buddy, so I can go lay down.*

He didn't budge. "Ma'am, where do you live?"

"In there." I pointed to the metal shop, and his curious gaze intensified.

"In there?"

"Yes, we have a little apartment . . ." I started to explain, until I realized how ridiculous I must look. Greasy, matted, bath-robed woman with a shovel and an egg. I put my head down and walked past Mr. Sheriff into our little condo and shut the door.

We love to entertain. There is nothing better than a party. The more people the better. Of course the initial challenge with the condo was the obvious lack of space. During the spring and summer evenings we barbecued outside. Rick would fire up the old, rickety *cue* he got for free somewhere. "I couldn't believe they were just going to throw this away. . ." We had an old picnic table, and when dusk settled in, our living-room lamp and an extension cord created the perfect ambiance. Winter was a little tougher, so the family was shocked to get *The Call.*

"Thanksgiving at the condo? Where will we sit?"

Their concern was cute, but we had it all figured out. "We can borrow a few tables from church and set them up in the shop, cook the turkey in the oven (that was strategically located next to the rack of pipe parts), and ask everyone to bring side dishes."

"You think that little fireplace will keep the place warm enough for them?"

"It'll be a beautiful day; we'll have a great time." It was and we did. My mom helped decorate the table, and if you didn't glance up to take in the surrounding tools, it looked nice. My aunt BJ, a favorite aunt from San Francisco, especially enjoyed the post-meal scenic stroll.

The area surrounding Volta actually is very pretty. Volta, by the way, is a little town just outside of Los Banos. There is probably a total of twenty houses grouped together to form a little community, and the condo was on the outer edge of town. Rosie's feed barn is the only proprietary establishment, and Rosie sells everything from animal feed to microwaveable sandwiches. She is quite a character and was one of the first *Voltaites* I met. Just beyond the cluster of small homes is wide-open expanse, mostly pastureland, bordered by foothills that separate us from the ocean and the cool breezes. Rick was affectionately called the mayor of Volta, since we owned a few homes out there.

When he got out of college, he knew he wanted to start his own business and own rental homes. The cheapest and only way he could get started was to purchase a piece of land in Volta, move in an old home, and set it up. This required a mountain of work. He ran water lines, dug septic tanks, watered the dirt until there was some grass to mow, and rented the place out. After the home was established, he went to the bank, took out a mortgage against it, bought another piece of dirt, and repeated the cycle. By the time we married, he was solidly established as a landlord.

We enjoyed walking through Volta and taking in the view of the foothills. We took a spin through the town and pointed out who lived in which house; each home had an interesting story. Then we headed out toward the hills to soak in the beauty. It truly was a memorable Thanksgiving Day.

Condo parties were, I must say, quite popular. We knew how to do it up. Our friends had formed a band, so we pulled in an old trailer and put some hay around the edge. They had a stage, and we had live entertainment. Another friend had horses; he brought his oldest nag over for kiddy rides. A horseshoe pit was constructed, and the competition was brutal. Swinging from the rafter in our carport, the most eligible lamb was butchered for the barbecue. And the party was on. Rick liked to cook lamb stew in a huge pot over an open fire . . . the parties were a hit. I discovered Los Banos had an abundance of fun, caring people. I hugely enjoyed my new friends.

I loved my job as a school nurse in Dos Palos, a small neighboring farming community. I had craved Pediatrics. I longed to work with kids. This was as close as I could get. The hours were good. I had weekends off, holidays off, and worked regular shifts. It wasn't too hard to kiss the hospital goodbye.

We were teased continuously, "Are you going to hang a hammock in the corner of your bedroom when your first kid is born? Hey, Howard, how many cribs can you fit out in the shop?" I was pregnant. We were deliriously happy and wondering if maybe it was time to move. Kurtis and Debbie had just moved out, and we longingly admired the 800-square foot palace next door. It was time.

Rick tore into the house in his usual flurry. I couldn't wait to get home each evening to see what progress he had made. He pulled up all the stinky carpets, exposing beautiful hardwood floors. The wall came down between the kitchen and living room, making one large living area, and the bathroom was gutted. He installed a beautiful woodstove in the living room and built brick and barn wood cabinets in the kitchen. A friend had just torn down a barn, so the wood was free. Rick had acquired a pile of bricks during another house demo, and the sink and faucets were in the shop. Guess what? The remodel was free, but beautiful. We actually bought a new bed, and I refinished Rick's grandmother's old kitchen table. He bought me two beautiful white couches for Christmas at a liquidation sale. "They're really high quality couches; you can barely see the water stain along the bottom edge" And they turned out to be one of our better bargains after we figured out how to re-stain them every year with blue RIT dye to cover all the stains our four kids would deposit on them. We had our first home.

We were being teased again. "Where you gonna put that fourth kid, Howard? They're already stacked like cordwood." We were a bit cramped. Joel and Kate had bunk beds, and Mallory's crib was wedged into the corner of the small bedroom. Rick had a solution. "Look, Honey, the front porch will be the foundation for the third bedroom."

Really. I eyed the small porch skeptically. A bedroom. . . His ideas just always seemed to work. Two weekends later, the little room was framed up and looked like it had always been there. New front steps were poured, and we had a 1,000-square-foot, three-bedroom home. We were ready for Bryce's arrival. The girls moved into the new room and the boys in the old room. The good news was that we had more space. The bad news was that I figured we might live in Volta the rest of our lives. Adventure was fun, but I still dreamed of a real house in town with a garage, sprinklers in the lawn, sidewalks, maybe even a pool.

It felt like we were the only English-speaking family in Volta. Our farming community has a high population of Hispanic farm workers. They are wonderful people, but I was especially tired of the way our neighbors chose to play their music. Their favorite blasting method was pulling the car on the front lawn, flopping the trunk open, and turning the music on as loud as the cheap, scratchy speakers could pound out. I grew weary of my surroundings.

We had continued to acquire properties and had recently purchased a "cash cow" trailer park. This dumpy place was a gold mine. It was also a ton of work for Rick to keep up. He had to be there several hours a day, and all day during the summer months when the migrant workers came to town. He also still had all the other properties and their upkeep. He was on overload.

We decided to build a new home. We looked at house plans and at property, but the process was painfully slow. Finally, one afternoon I called a realtor and asked her to drive me around and show me available homes in town. I didn't care for any I looked at but pointed out a two-story ranch-style home with a porch. "That's the country style we like." The next day Sally called, "Sandy, I knocked on the door of that cute house you liked last night. The people are interested in selling." My heart soared. Our dream home, available . . . the negotiation was Rick's worst nightmare. He was a mess. I had learned to stay neutral when we looked at any property, thereby maintaining a negotiating edge. He always said, "There's not any property I have to have. Don't ever act like you like it; always point out the flaws." But I had fallen in love with a house, and he wanted desperately to buy it. They knew it, and we knew it. He had lost his edge. He was a nervous wreck. He paced, he fumed. It was the first home he would buy without a rental income. We would have to pay the mortgage. It was almost too much for him. God worked out the details. We were even able to purchase the empty lot next door, which we would later incorporate into the backyard. Automatic garage doors, sprinklers in the lawn, sidewalk, garbage disposal, dishwasher . . . it even had a pool.

*T*

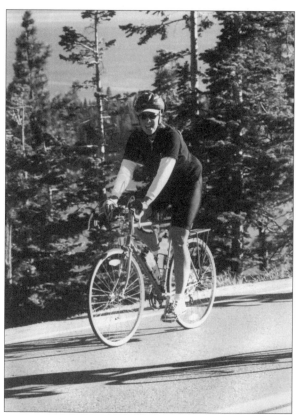

*Cruising around Lake Tahoe.*

# The Blasting Continues: Chemo Two

Before each treatment, I prayed for God to show me someone he wanted me to talk to, and I always met someone interesting. As Rick sat faithfully holding my hand, we would chat with our cubicle companions. Harriet was a classy-looking lady in her smart wool skirt and blazer. She was working at a laptop. With her matching wool hat, she looked the part of the efficient businesswoman. "My name is Sandy. You look wonderful. What kind of therapy are you receiving?"

She explained how she had been treated for breast cancer two years ago. She was fine for a year "but I couldn't get rid of a nagging cough." The cancer had metastasized to her lungs. Now she was receiving a chemotherapeutic agent called Herceptin to keep the tumor from growing. Every three months she had an x-ray, and if the tumor had not grown, she and her husband celebrated. She still managed to work part time for the city of San Jose, even though one out of the three weeks she was very sick. Listening to her story was horrifying, my worst nightmare sitting next to me. I wanted to cry for me, for her. I wanted to hug her, pray for her, but I didn't want to look at her with that "Oh-you-poor-thing" look that I so often received. Instead I stared straight ahead, saying and doing nothing. I think of Harriet often.

People's reactions toward me were one of the most fascinating aspects of cancer. Their stares, uncomfortable glances, the Oh-you-poor-thing look, overreacting, or just plain ignoring me—turning and walking the other way like I was contagious. I experienced them all, and I could empathize with all of them. What do you say? How do you react when a friend or loved one is in crisis? There is no correct answer. Some days I craved the hugs and empathy; other days, that same reaction by a well-meaning friend was loathed. "Leave me alone; don't feel sorry for me. Just treat me like you've always treated me!" I would silently scream. But the most appreciated responses, whether they said what I wanted to hear or not, were those based in love. When you're in crisis, all systems are on hyper alert. I could always sense the love and concern people conveyed. Most certainly, I could sense the scared, threatened people. I understood I was their Harriet. I was their worst nightmare staring them in the face. Several women disappeared from my life during this time. I never saw them, and I knew they didn't want to see me. I understood.

Back to love, react to people in crisis with love. It doesn't matter exactly what you say or do; what will be felt is love.

"Hey, some of us are going to ride our bikes around Lake Tahoe, wanna come?" My friend Dana plopped on our couch and gushed on about this "fun," seventy-five-mile bike ride.

"You're nuts, absolutely nuts." I had been a moderate exercise enthusiast for all of my life. After my high-school sports career ended, I continued jogging on a semi-regular basis and swam regularly. I enjoyed working out and started thinking the bike-riding thing might be kinda fun. "Maybe I'll give it a whirl." On a neighbor's borrowed ten-speed, I joined Dana on a ride into the country, a little fifteen-mile spin. Heck, we could talk and joke around and see a lot more country than when going on my little three-mile jogs. I liked it. Maybe this seventy-five-mile ride was doable!

Four months and many miles later, we completed the ride around Lake Tahoe. It was one of the most exciting days of my life. What a feeling of accomplishment and satisfaction. I felt that I had truly enjoyed one of God's most beautiful creations up close and personal. I had seen firsthand how the emerald green of the lake's edge extended around the entire lake. The smell of pine trees, the home with hundreds of daffodils in the front yard, the camaraderie of fellow cyclists—I totally enjoyed every aspect. I was hooked. Since I had added biking, a triathlon was the next logical step. To be able to participate in the tri at New Melones Dam in August became my goal, and God provided the way. It turned out that the event was at the tail end of treatment number two, so I was still feeling pretty darn good. I was ready to go.

We had the tradition of camping out at New Melones Dam for the weekend. Some of us did the tri individually; some of our friends formed teams. We didn't care; we were just having fun. Now, picture a rolling desert with a dam poured into one of the valleys, and that's where we camped. Right in the dirt. There were about thirty of us hanging out, including all of the kids, and we had a great time. The kids brought their bikes, roller blades, and scooters to take advantage of the hills. The adults ate, drank, and socialized. One of our friends was a master with the Dutch oven and CarolAnn kept cranking out gourmet meals. Rick was in heaven. Chili, baked chickens, cobbler, we had it all. Saturday morning all the participants were up early to eat our dried oatmeal, which is supposed to taste good when it's reconstituted. We loaded our bikes in the trucks and headed for the starting line.

The first leg of a tri is the swim. I was especially fond of the swim. Besides enjoying swimming, when I had my cap on, I felt completely normal. The swim is made more exciting by the totally chaotic start. A few hundred swimmers smashed together waiting for the gun to go off, and then the real thrashing began. We always wait for the red hots to take off before we go. Still, there is a moderate amount of body bumping, something I oddly find exhilarating. My oldest son, Joel, was with us—in the beginning anyway. He is a competitive swimmer and finished near the front of the pack. Rick was also with us, in his kayak. He's our faithful personal lifeguard.

After the swim comes the run up the boat ramp to the bikes. I hesitated before I jumped on my bike. I remember Mallory standing there with my scarf. I had to pull off my cap, but didn't want my baldness exposed. "Mom, just pull it off!"

"But Mal…"

"Mom, just pull it off!"

The bike section is a total blast. It is sixteen miles of rolling hills, with riders encouraging each other along the way. It's so fun to see all the different bikes and different sizes and shapes of people who choose to compete. There are, of course, the serious athletes with perfect bodies, looking to better their times, and a surprising number of older people like us, just having fun. Pre-race preparations involve printing one's age on one's calf with permanent ink. There's a great deal of satisfaction in passing a younger person, and admiration when a sixty-year old woman blazes by!

Rick is also our personal mechanic. He drives his truck slowly along the course, offering encouragement, drinks, and any mechanical support necessary. The kids ride in the back of the truck yelling and cheering. The whole event is quite festive. Until the run. Off on an isolated cross-country course, it is hot, dry, and dusty. No cheering, just hot, sweaty, grunting bodies. While my friend Dana anticipates this portion and lopes happily along, I am among the grunting. Four miles later, we emerge to cross the finish line. And this was an extra special finish. I was exhilarated and so thankful to be healthy enough to participate. I gave Rick a big sweaty hug. Thank you, Lord, for your blessings.

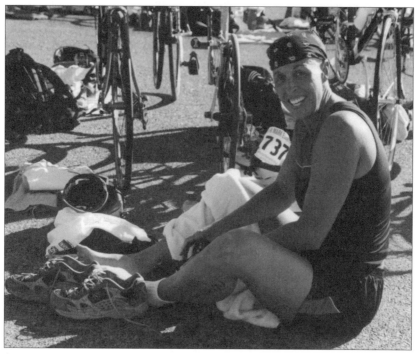

*Getting ready for the bike ride at New Melones Triathlon.*

# The Worst of the Blast: Chemo Three

Back in the Infusion Room for number three. Getting used to this—getting psyched up for one week of very sick, one week of slightly sick, and one week of pretty good. Ignorance truly is bliss.

They gave meds before and during the infusion, so the sickness didn't hit for three to four hours post treatment. On the way home, we stopped for a Jamba Juice. I love smoothies. We did some shopping and headed home. One hour after arriving home the vomiting started. The Jamba Juice was the first thing out. It was absolutely uncontrollable. I couldn't get comfortable in any place or position. For some reason I wanted to be outside. I made my way from the backyard to the front, dry heaving every few minutes, and ended on the bench on the front porch. Kate and Mallory brought big pillows for me, and Bryce reappeared with a pink teddy bear he had won at the fair. He placed it on my chest.

I hated the fear and concern I could see in their eyes. I felt like I was torturing them, but I couldn't stop. Rick called Stanford, "My wife is vomiting and can't stop. . ."

"What treatment did she just receive?"

"Number three."

"Oh, you'd better get her to your local hospital; number three is usually the roughest round." God had a plan for the emergency room. When we arrived, it was packed. Standing room only. We both experienced a moment of panic. Rick explained to the receptionist that Stanford had been notified of my condition and would be calling with orders. She graciously moved us to the front of the line, where we immediately met our triage nurse, a friendly, open-faced redheaded man named Kelvin.

"We don't have any beds, but you're not going to wait. I'm going to put you on a bed in the hall and start an IV right away." As he led me down the hall, I remember thinking how ironic it was that I was wearing my "Life is good" swimmer shirt. "But life really is good," I remember thinking. We are allowed to go through suffering as a process to draw us closer to Him. As I Peter 4 says, "Think of your sufferings as a weaning from that old sinful habit of always expecting to get you own way. Then you'll be able to live out your days free to pursue what God wants instead of being tyrannized by what you want."

"So do what you need to do. Lord, I just hope it's fast." Kelvin started the IV on the first stick. This was truly a blessing, since I was so dehydrated. It took a couple of hours for the nausea to abate, but during that time, Kelvin and Rick had an amazing talk. Seems that he was a traveling nurse who had just moved his family to Los Banos. His wife home-schooled their kids and was seeking to connect with Christian women. They had been visiting churches in the community but hadn't found a church home yet. Several of the moms in my Bible study were also home-school moms. We exchanged phone numbers, and the following week we met his darling southern wife, Sarah. She attended weekly and networked with the other home-schoolers. Before they moved back to Mississippi the following year, Sarah related that she and Kelvin had been praying the very morning that Kelvin and I met in the ER for a group of friends in Los Banos to connect with Sarah. Even in the midst of suffering, we could see God moving.

# The Blast Changes: Chemo Four

There was no more ignorance. I knew how brutal the side effects could be, and subconsciously my system shut down. My body was not going to allow any more of this poison in. They wrapped my arms in hot pads; I hung my arm down, pumped my fist, thought positive thoughts, pumped some more fist, nothing. My body was shut down, the poison locked out. Finally, three nurses and eight sticks later, I had an IV. Treatment number four was on the way. I was nauseated just sitting there waiting for the inevitable red juice. Two seconds into the push and I was thoroughly nauseated and totally ill. Was this all in my head?

My oncologist told a story of his colleague who, while skiing one day, saw a former patient of his. He skied up to her to say hello and she threw up on his skis. Physical or emotional, the nausea was very real.

Thankfully, our latest report was very positive. The tumor had shrunk significantly. Rick was elated. The appointment was immediately prior to my infusion, so my enthusiasm was tempered with dread. "I want to see you after your chemo, just to make sure your reaction is not as severe as last time," Dr. Carmon droned on. With the big mustache and eyes hidden behind glasses, the only connection I had formed with my oncologist was one of sickness and puking. I dreaded our appointments. He and Rick developed a camaraderie with one another. I left the small talk to my husband. I was happy to sit quietly in the corner. I tried to imagine if I had met Carmon in a different setting if I would have liked him, but I could not remove myself far enough from the situation to even speculate on that thought.

My husband is very tall and very fun. At 5'10", I was always attracted to tall men. I knew I'd hit the jackpot when Rick sauntered into the room and flopped on the beanbag in the corner. I would later learn that he is 6'7". Next to him, I feel quite petite. My college roommate had taken a teaching job in Los Banos and invited me to a Back to School teachers' party. "You're going to meet your husband! I've got the perfect guy for you!" Boy was she right. We hit it off the very first night. It was evident from the greetings he received as he entered the room that he was well respected and loved. I was very intrigued with this gentle giant and happily discovered that he could also dance!

We had a blast dancing in Ron's little kitchen with the stereo blasting out scratchy rock 'n roll tunes. I knew this was a special man, and I soon learned the way to Rick's heart was truly through his stomach. The man loved to eat; it was his hobby. While I recalled life's meaningful events by people I met, or what I was wearing, Rick remembered people and places by the food he ate. "Oh yeah, I remember her. She makes great apple pie! . . . Yeah, that's a cool city; there's a restaurant with a great rack of lamb."

True to character, Rick associates Stanford, along with the obvious pain and discomfort, with great macaroon cookies and homemade, cheap breakfasts. We made a habit of leaving home early on appointment days to avoid the Bay Area traffic and to eat breakfast in the cafeteria while we waited. He could choose from a dazzling array of fresh baked goods and enticing special foods. While we waited for Dr. Carmon, Rick munched one of the huge, chocolate-dipped macaroon cookies. "Looks like this round is going to be much easier," Dr. Carmon announced after he had poked around for a while. "Next four rounds will be a different drug. This drug doesn't make you nauseous; it has a sort of flu-like effect on people." A satisfying array of cuss words floated through my head as I glared at this man. "The tumor is definitely shrinking; keep up the good work!" He and Rick finished with some pleasant chatter. All I could think of was getting to the car and getting home.

I came home to a clean house. While we were gone, my mom and dad, in-laws, and six friends cleaned our home from top to bottom. What an amazing blessing that was. God told me He loved me through His people. Not only did I have a clean house, I was emotionally and spiritually lifted. Meals poured in all week from our wonderful and faithful friends. Kate became my secret angel. When I got up, my coffee was made. When I went to bed, my covers were turned down. Loving touches surrounded me. Dana sent her girls over, and along with Mallory, they set up a luxury bath. Candles, music, chocolates, lemon-ice water, chamber music playing softly in the background. It was an event and so incredibly relaxing. God's people were rallying again, and it was a beautiful sight

Treatment five was difficult. The new side effects included severe body aches for the first week, mouth sores, extreme fatigue, and an ulcer. The week following the treatment, I went to work and sat at my desk. It was 8 a.m., and I was exhausted. I realized the folly of what I was trying to do. I would use what little energy I had to slog through the day and do half as much as I should, come home, and go to bed. I needed to be expending what little energy I had on my family. But taking a leave of absence from work felt like giving in to the cancer. As if it would win a round if I did. And I desperately did not want to give in, not one single round. I started to cry as I understood what I had to do. I called our nurse coordinator, Leslie, and explained my situation. "I'm so sorry, but I can't do it any more. I need to take a leave of absence until my treatment is done." She was wonderful, as were my principal and staff. I managed not to cry until I got outside, when I was consumed with sobs and total sadness.

"Why are you so upset? Think of this is a long vacation." But I felt like I had just handed off one of my kids for safekeeping, shunned my responsibility, given in to the cancer. I cried all the way home and then some. But it was definitely the best move I could have made.

Despite all the help and encouragement, I was feeling alone. I cried out to God, "Are you there? Do you care?" I was battling an ongoing case of insomnia. Despite my constant fatigue, I had been unable to fall asleep naturally following my diagnosis back in July. Bedtime brought anxiety and worry. When would I fall asleep? How many pills would it take? Often when I lay down and closed my eyes, my heart would race in anxiety. I felt like a spiritual failure, because I couldn't pray myself out of this anxiety.

The week after treatment number five, I was preparing my Sunday school lesson. It happened to be on the subject of worry and included the verse in Matthew, "Why should you worry? He cares for the sparrows. Have faith, trust God." Turns out that it was the wrong lesson, but I was thankful God had showed me the verse I needed. I ended up whipping together a lesson on temptation at the last minute that was equally encouraging. The book of Deuteronomy has the good Jews wandering in the desert crying out to the Lord, "Why have you abandoned us?" He had just sent manna, and already they were crying and complaining that they felt abandoned and alone. "Wow. That's me," I thought. "He keeps blessing me and caring for me, and here I am crying already for more." And in His time He sends manna. He was answering me, quite clearly.

Nonetheless, I was still down and tired. Emotionally, physically, spiritually tired. Tired of feeling sick. Tired of aching bones and muscles, and tired of headaches; tired of numb hands and feet. Sick and tired from being tired, I had absolutely no energy, none. One night I cried just thinking about what it would be like to ride my bike again and be healthy. To be able to ride as hard as I wanted, feel the wind in my face, sweat, feel strong again. It would be glorious. Then came my lowest day. A near debilitating side effect of this chemo was the numbing of my hands and feet. It hurt to walk, and holding anything in my hands was painful. I was developing an ulcer; the stomach pain increased. I had to surrender to the couch.

One Monday my mission for the day was to get to the bus stop at t 2 p.m. to pick up Bryce. By 10 o'clock, I conceded that I was not going to be able to do it. I called my local GP and explained the pain; she generously offered to bring some ulcer medicine by the house. I also had pain medication at the pharmacy that needed to be picked up. Rick was gone for the day, and I was unable to contact him. I called Laura and her husband Bob, a local pastor, to do a pharmacy run for me. I spent a good deal of the day on the couch crying in frustration and pain. Like the Israelites, I felt abandoned by God, even though he had just given me manna the day before. I feared I would never get better, that the cancer was going to slowly rot me away. I was totally wiped out. Word spread; friends rallied and started coming by to encourage me. God spoke through His people again.

Laura and Bob had been in Los Banos for three years; he was the pastor at a local church. We met through swim team and became fast friends. Bob had helped me immensely in my Christian walk. I had been raised in church, but did not hear and understand the Gospel message until I was eighteen and invited to a different church. The pastor clearly explained how Jesus had died for our sins. "For God so loved the world that He gave His only begotten son, that whoever believes in Him should not perish but have everlasting life." - John 3:16.

I believed that Jesus had died for me, but the concept of God was that of some big foreign power in the sky. And I knew I didn't want to get on His bad side. The pastor explained that man is sinful, "For all have sinned and fallen short of the glory of God." - Romans 3:23. I didn't have a problem with that either. I knew I did some bad stuff, but overall, I was a good person. I was set. Then he clarified the concept and penalty of sin, "For the wages of sin is death, but the gift of God is eternal life in Christ Jesus our Lord." - Romans 6:23. Now I was interested. I had never really considered the permanence of Hell and Heaven. And the beautiful simplicity of God's offer of a guaranteed ticket to heaven: "For whoever calls upon the name of the Lord shall be saved." Romans 10:13.

I was impressed with this information and felt a sense of urgency to ensure my eternal destination. I asked Jesus into my heart that morning and joined a Bible study. I had never read or studied the Bible and was fascinated to learn of the immensity of God's love for me. I vowed to live my life to please Him. I carried out my Christian life in fits and starts since that time. When I met Rick, I knew he was the kindest man I had ever met, but his propensity for foul language led me to believe he wasn't where I hoped he would be spiritually. I had decided not to date men who were not Christian. After the second date, I asked if we could talk.

"Sure, but there's something I want to ask you, too. You go first."

I explained how important my faith in God was to me, and my desire to date men with the same beliefs. I asked him where he was spiritually.

"Wow, that's so weird. That's exactly what I wanted to ask you about," he explained. He had sensed something different about me and wanted to know more about it. He related how he had not been raised in a church, and Sundays were strictly another workday on his parents' horse ranch in Los Banos. He explained how his younger brother went to church with a friend to get out of the work at home and to eat the donuts that were served. Rick resented the fact that he stayed home to work while his brother loped off. Because of this, he generally resented the church. He went on to explain that he had recently met the financial goals he had set for himself, the goals he had always believed would bring total contentment and fulfillment. But now he knew there was more to it. There was still a sense of something unsatisfied and unfulfilled in him, and he didn't know how fix it.

We sat on my old green couch and talked more about Jesus, about His amazing sacrifice and love for us. I showed him the verses that had meant so much to me, gave him my Bible, and then in thought he drove away. Two days later he called and excitedly explained that he finally "got it," too. He had asked Jesus into his heart and knew he had found the key to contentment and fulfillment. He had found his real purpose in life.

Even though I knew my purpose in life was to "love God and glorify Him," I consistently felt I failed at this task more often than I succeeded. I was often frustrated in my Christian walk. Pastor Bob helped me immensely in this area, when he explained the two common sense questions I could easily ask to turn a conversation toward the spiritual realm. What is your spiritual background, and where are you on your spiritual journey? These questions provided an easy avenue in which I could share my faith, explore the other person's spiritual needs, and open the door to inviting them to study scriptures with me. And to my delight, Bob even provided basic Bible studies explaining basic foundational Biblical truths. I was shocked to find how many people enjoyed talking about their faith, or lack of it, and how they had arrived at that place. I found that my frustration level decreased when I could comfortably share my faith with others. The padlock had been cut off; I felt spiritually free to confidently go where God led. I was fulfilling my purpose.

The morning after my lowest day, I woke at 4 a.m. and felt no pain. Slowly I sat up to evaluate. My hands and feet felt good, stomach good . . . how can this be? I woke up Rick. "I don't hurt! Dear God, I don't hurt!" It was my first miracle. The following morning I went for a mile jog; OK, still feeling good, "Am I cured, healed?" I ran in the house and showered. I still felt good; I had energy. "Thank you, Lord!" At the grocery store, I told the clerk about my miracle. I ran all the errands that had been piling up, and I told everyone who would listen about my miracle. "Dare I even think it? Was I healed?" That night our family went out to dinner to celebrate my pain-free, energy-filled day.

What a blessed gift it had been. The next day proved it had been a pure gift from God, a respite in the storm, because I crashed. I crashed hard. All the old symptoms were back. Yet emotionally, spiritually, I was refreshed, ready to continue the battle. Thank you, Lord, for sending the manna.

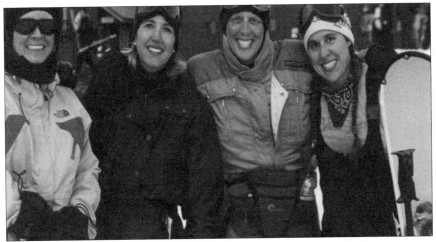

*Laura, Dana, me, and Renee on our amazing ski day.*

# More Manna

I love to ski. Dana and Laura love to ski, so naturally we do an annual ski trip. This is a women-only event, and it is a blast. Laura is a phenomenal skier, like those people on TV who swish effortlessly and beautifully down any terrain. I am a chug boat; I do my best to keep up with them.

Our trip had been scheduled for the following week. It became my top worry. I wouldn't be able to keep up, and I didn't want to slow them down or ruin their trip. Should I stay home? Should I go and sit in the lodge? If I sit in the lodge, would I wear my hat and look like I was ready to head out at any minute? Or wear my scarf and look sick, yet comfortable, or the wig and be itchy? These are the things a bald woman contemplates.

They proposed a compromise of leaving home later in the day and skiing a half day Wednesday and a full day Thursday. The thought of driving up, not having my nap, and skiing all afternoon was very scary, but I couldn't stay home.

I felt great; it was unfathomable that I could have so much energy. It was a pure grace thing. I was a bundle of energy and speed. I went full blast all afternoon on no nap, amazingly. I couldn't believe it. Back at the hotel, we relaxed in the Jacuzzi before going out to dinner. Up early, we skied all day Thursday, and I still felt great. It was my best day skiing ever, because I totally appreciated every moment. I was in awe that my body was actually able to ski, and totally and completely amazed by God's grace. He had delivered manna again.

Followed by *the crash*. Since insomnia continued to haunt me, every night was a frustration of exhaustion and inability to sleep. This Friday night I cried uncontrollably as Rick held me. It felt like when I was pregnant, when I would cry for no reason and was just unable to stop. I was absolutely exhausted, yet unable to fall asleep. I hated taking sleeping pills, but I kept thinking of what one of the nurses had told me, "Just get through this, and then worry about stopping the medicines." That bit of advice really comforted me. Rick was his usual supportive, compassionate self, and eventually we fell asleep.

I was totally dreading my last treatment. I absolutely did not want to go. I really did not want to go, not at all. I presented my case to Rick. "I'm thinking maybe I should not get this last round." He lay down on the bed next to me, and we discussed the pros and cons for a time. After Rick got in the shower, I laid there, cried, and prayed. I wanted to do the right thing for my family but hoped that maybe we could figure a way around this thing. Toweling off, he asked, "Remember when you first got sick, what you told me?"

I said, "Don't worry about me, whatever it is, I can take it."

"Yeah, you did. And you have. You're almost done, Honey, just one more." Interestingly I felt relieved that he had encouraged me to finish, because I truly did want to finish. I didn't want to have any regrets later. I also felt loved, because I knew he really hated to see me suffer. But I knew his greatest desire was for me to live. And, lastly, I felt anger that he would encourage me to do something that made me feel so sick.

I did postpone my last chemo for one week so I could attend our friends' wedding. By then I was four weeks post-treatment seven and feeling pretty darn good for the beautiful event. We danced all night and had a wonderful time. I had my wig on, and except for my crinkled toenails and fingernails, I looked pretty normal. We had a family picture taken that night, and I kept thinking how amazing it was that I could look and feel so good. Yet I knew that in three days I would be back on the couch. But it was the last round! "Will this ever really be over? What will it be like to have a 'normal' life again?" I was filled with relief and dread.

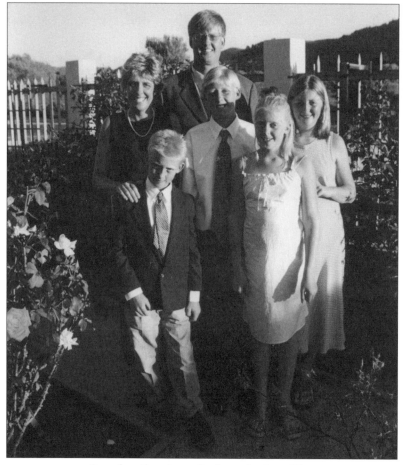

## 11

*Our family photo before the last blast*

# The Last Blast

On January 28, 2003, I walked out of infusion therapy for the last time. I waved goodbye to a couple of nurses, but no huge goodbyes. I was not really attached to anyone, since I had been assigned different nurses for each treatment. I was so excited just to get the heck out of there and never, ever, ever go back.

I couldn't wait for the poison to be out of my body, to have energy again, to ride my bike, and to feel strong. The simple things I used to take for granted, like blow-drying my hair, not wearing makeup because I had my own eyebrows and lashes, not wearing a hat . . . the end was so close. Just a little more time on the couch.

A couple of weeks later I came up for air. It was over. I had survived chemotherapy, and the tumor had shrunk enough for a lumpectomy. This was exhilarating news.

During my nurses training, I remember working with a couple of mastectomy patients who were bemoaning the loss of their breast. "Get over it, I thought . . . Move on, at least you're alive." I always assumed that the loss of a body part, especially a "useless" breast was not a big deal. "Just suck it up and move on."

Not so. When faced with the very real prospect of losing my breast, I was extremely concerned. Obviously if it was the breast or me, whack away. But, if at all possible, to avoid losing it, I wanted to follow that path. The news that the tumor had shrunk to a manageable size was elating. The chemo had been worth it. Now just surgery and radiation remained, and I was through with this journey!

On surgery morning, I saw Dr. Denis in the hallway and stopped to say hi. "Hey, Dr. Denis, how are you doing today?" I cheerfully addressed him. Poor man. We had spoken over the phone several times, but he had not seen me for three months. I recognized the blank look on his face. There had been many times in the last nine months when I had walked right by people I knew well. They had no idea who I was, until sometimes the blank look cleared. They would figure out who I was and then the usual, "Oh, Sandy! How are you?" I knew Denis was thinking, "Uh, which pasty white, skinny bald woman is this?" I wondered how many breast surgery cases he had that day. I figured we all looked about the same on the operating table.

He truly was one of the many, many committed professionals I met at Stanford. It wasn't unusual for him to return my calls at 9:30 or 10:00 at night. He obviously works incredibly long, exhausting days. I am so thankful for all the kind, dedicated, and efficient medical professionals I met. From Janelle, who schedules appointments in an amazingly kind and accommodating manner, to Trina, the darling Irish nurse coordinator with her sweet, compassionate brogue. I was in awe of these wonderful people who performed emotionally and physically exhausting work day after day.

Back in the hallway, Dr. Denis pretended to know who I was. I encouraged him to "cut a wide girth" around my tumor. He promised he would. It would be the only time I saw him that day. Post surgically, he spoke with Rick to deliver the news that my lymph system was clear. The chemo had done its job. Rick was crying as he came alongside my gurney and grabbed my hand. I knew it was good news— he looked so happy. Something about lymph, clear. Amazingly, I was not overjoyed. It was a small positive step, but I wanted *all* the cancer out, all of it, and I couldn't let down my guard to rejoice over this good news.

Apparently I was allergic to the anesthesia, because I spent the next twelve hours vomiting. By morning I was totally wiped. I was crumpled in my bed as the morning-shift nurse came breezing into the room. "Good morning, Mr. Howard. How are you this morning?"

"Oh, dear God, she thinks I'm a man." I was too stunned to speak. I stared blankly at the poor lady, who, realizing her mistake, tried to backtrack. She glanced down at my chart, "I'm so sorry, Mrs. Howard, and can I get anything for you?"

"I want to go home." And I wanted a picture of the real me and my family by my bed so nurses and doctors could see who I really was and would be again.

Part of my husband's charm is his absolute down to earth nature. He drives a beat up truck, spends most of his day in dirty work clothes, and is as friendly to strangers as he is to his best friends. At 6'7", he is the tallest man in town. He is a recognizable guy. Sometimes when I spot him uptown, I will sit at a distance and watch in admiration. In his booming voice he greets everyone he encounters with, "How are you today?" shakes hands, and genuinely listens when people talk to him. Rick has excelled in everything he has done in life by sheer hard work and determination. And, he is extremely thrifty. He prides himself on never buying a shirt that costs more than five dollars. His idea of a perfect day is going to his ranch, checking fences, and doctoring cows. Part of his unpretentious manner includes the complete shunning of modern technology. He operates his business with a handheld solar calculator, and a cell phone is

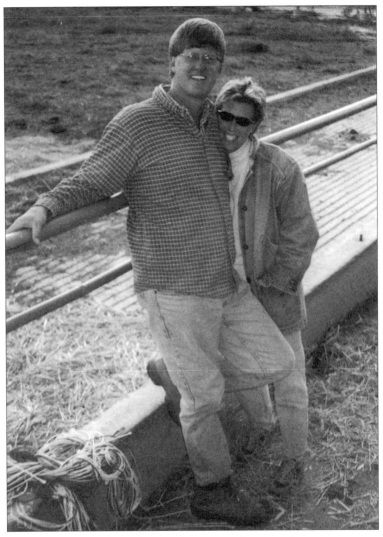

*Rick and me relaxing at the ranch.*

out of the question. So it was on a borrowed cell phone that I finally spoke with Dr Denis.

It had been a very long week post surgically as we waited for the call telling us if they got all the cancer. We wanted to attend the annual Yosemite Farm Credit dinner in Turlock, but we didn't want to miss "The Call." I borrowed Dana's cell, and on the way home, 10 at night, it finally rang. "Ah, yes. Sandy, this is Fred Denis, Stanford Medical Center."

"Yeah, Fred," I thought, "I gotcha, just relax and give me the goods."

I said, "Hi, Fred, thanks for calling. Is this workday about over for you?"

"Well, actually, I have a few more phone calls to make."

"Great," I'm thinking, "how many other women are in my shoes tonight?" Better keep this conversation short so the others can hear their news tonight. "So, what did you figure out, did you get it all?"

"Well, at this point it appears that there are undifferentiated cells at the margin of the excision."

"That's bad," I thought.

"Well, we do not have a margin of clean tissue."

"That definitely sounds bad." He was saying that the edges of the tumor had cancer cells, and they needed a strip of tissue around the cut-out chunk that had no cancer cells, referred to by cancer guys as *clear margins*. My margins weren't clear. (I still have cancer growing in me.) "So, Fred, what you're saying is, you didn't get it all and you need to cut more out, is that correct?"

He rambled on some more about cells being in the wrong place, which meant they just weren't positive they got it all. I wanted positive. "Fred, you need to cut more out, right?"

"Yes, that would be a good choice." The surgery couldn't be scheduled for two more weeks. My final surgery date was still two weeks away. I had two more weeks of lugging cancer around in my body. I couldn't wait to get it out. Totally out.

Two days before my final surgery Rick came home from work and dashed upstairs. To my horror, I could hear him vomiting in the bathroom. He flopped on the bed groaning, "Honey, you have to get out of here. You can't get sick." We discussed our limited options, made some phone calls and decided I would move out for two days to be as far from his germs as possible. I hated the decision, but knew it had to be done. Bob and Laura had a spare bedroom in their home, so I moved in. Laura drove me to Stanford the next day. They had promised a quick in and out surgery, and with a change in the anesthesia to ward off the post-surgery nausea, I was discharged and home late the same night. I couldn't wait to get home and hold Rick, who was finally feeling better. Now we just had to wait five days for the pathology report.

I had gone to drop the kids off at school, buzzed over to Wal-Mart, got the oil changed in my Suburban, came home, and Rick met me in the garage to help carry the bags in. Receipt books for Rick, a box to mail my burned pan back to the manufacturer, Capri suns for lunches, basic items of life I will remember forever. I sat the bags down and turned to go out for more when Rick stopped me. He gave me a huge hug. "Trina called, and they got it all this time. There was no cancer in the part they just took out."

I froze and held onto him. My mind was racing, trying to process that information. I was afraid to let myself believe he really said "they got it all," in case it was somehow wrong information. "She said they got it all?"

"They got it all."

"They got it all?"

"Honey, they got it all. It's gone." The sobbing started slowly and built rapidly. Rick led me over to the couch and held me as I finally let it all out. I felt completely out of control. If the roof had caved in, I would not have been able to move or stop crying. Mallory was home sick from school that day, and she came down the stairs to see what all the racket was about. She thought I was hysterically laughing and was shocked to find me crying. She sat on the couch next to Rick and they settled in to watch me cry. Thirty minutes later, I was concerned this might go on for hours. I really wanted to call my parents and our friends with the news, but I couldn't talk. For nine months I had told myself to suck it up, don't cry, be tough. Now I didn't have to any longer. It was finally over, and the floodgates had opened. An hour later, I was finally able to call my parents, but after I told them, the crying started all over again. I made several more phone calls and finally collapsed exhausted on my bed. I thought, "This is the first time I've laid on my bed in nine months without cancer. This is the first time I've brushed my teeth without cancer." Life became BC and AC (Before Cancer and After Cancer). The cancer was actually gone.

# 12

# Craniosacral What?

Unfortunately, the insomnia raged on. I had hoped that once the cancer was gone, my insomnia might give it up, let go, let me be. Not so. As I began radiation treatment, the frustrating nights continued. Usually by midnight, I gave up on relaxation and praying and took a pill that, I hoped, would knock me out. Sometimes it did, sometimes it didn't.

The day after a sleepless night was frustrating and exhausting. I was frightened this might become a lifetime affliction, and that was a terrifying thought. What was causing it? Do I have a physical malfunction? Is it the chemo left in my system? Is it another disease? I asked Dr. Carmon to refer me to the Stanford Sleep Disorders Center, but the appointment was still three months away.

Meantime, radiation was a breeze, a fascinating phenomenon of technical wizardry. I loved asking questions each session. The process was truly amazing. A new cancer facility had just been completed in Merced; it was handily located across the street from my old friend, the Merced College pool. I scheduled my appointments for 11:30 a.m. so I could catch the public swim hour, swim some laps, and then head home. My swims had taken on an almost spiritual feel. I felt like the water was flushing all the poison out of my body. I was slowly feeling stronger. Swimming was exhilarating and refreshing, and, of course, the ultimate benefit was, with my cap on, I felt conspicuously inconspicuous. I also hoped the daily workouts would ease the insomnia, but exhausted as I was each night, I still could not fall asleep naturally.

My dear friend Shelly told me about something she had tried. It was called Craniosacral Therapy.

"What the heck is that?"

"It's some kind of energy thing. I don't know, it's very strange. When Lila held her hands over my chest, I felt like a weight had been lifted off my chest. My asthma didn't bother me; I could breathe normally."

Now, Shelly is a levelheaded Christian woman whom I deeply admire. During my treatment, she had called weekly and stopped by often to encourage me and to pray. "An energy thing?" I would normally snort and move on; after all, I was trained in Western medicine, and anything with a new age flair hinted of voodoo and satanism to me. I wanted nothing to do with it. "Maybe she can help you with your sleeping?" I was just desperate enough. Nothing else had worked, and I would not take pills for the rest of my life. Maybe if I just give it a try. I decided to call this Lila lady, to see if this cranial thing could help me.

"Yes, it can help with insomnia," her gentle, calm, voice assured me. "Remember, it's not a magic cure; it can be a long process, but it may be able to help you."

At $55 a whack, I thought, this better help fast. Her salon was a haven in the otherwise small, unremarkable farming town of Dos Palos. Classical music was playing; I could hear water tinkling in the background, and it smelled so good. There were candles all around; it just felt cozy and safe. Back in a quiet room with clouds painted on the ceiling, I skeptically climbed up on the massage table. For ninety minutes she placed her hands gently on my feet and finally on my head. I tried to be open minded, not to laugh. "How the heck is this going to help me sleep?"

Lila patiently explained the concept of energy, and blockages. She explained that these blockages could be created through both physical and emotional trauma. "An emotional trauma can affect you as much or more than a physical trauma. The energy enters the body, and if the body does not process the influx of energy, it can get stuck. Eventually this excess energy forms what's known as an *energy cyst*, which blocks normal energy flow and can cause a variety of physical symptoms. This process, strange as it seems, gives the body energy to heal itself, energy to release these blockages."

"Including insomnia?"

"Absolutely. Your body will heal itself in layers, layers like those of an onion. There's no way to know in which layer the insomnia is lodged. Remember, it's a process."

A process, *in due time,* my whole cancer journey had become a process, a journey of revelation, understanding, and patience. . . "in due time." I was used to this concept now. I was developing patience.

I couldn't imagine that this soft-spoken petite woman could cure my insomnia by barely touching my body, but I lay back and relaxed and prayed. "Lord, if you've really sent me here, please work through this kind woman and allow my body to heal." As she sat behind me with her hands gently touching my head, I wisecracked, "What are you doing back there? Figuring out what you're going to fix for dinner tonight?"

She burst out in laughter. "No, no, I'm not thinking about dinner. I'm listening to your body."

This lady is definitely whacked, I conceded. But I didn't have any other options on the horizon, so I continued to lie there. "At least it's relaxing," I thought.

At the end of the session, she enthusiastically informed me that I had had several "good releases."

"That's a good thing?"

"Yes, that's a very good thing."

"Will I be able to sleep?"

"I don't know when you'll be able to sleep. Remember your body will release in layers. I don't know where the sleep disorder will be in that process."

I wanted to trust her; I needed hope, but I would not expose myself to any treatment that could have satanic influence. "There are two powers at work in the world, and probably some people in this work are fueled by the dark power," she explained. "I rely on God's power, the Holy Spirit, to guide me in my work. I am a tool, an instrument that He can use. I open myself for Him to work through me. I can make you no guarantees."

I truly wanted to believe this kind, Christian woman could help me; but it was all so out *there*.

"Look, I know you're skeptical, so I'll give you four free sessions. If you don't see any progress after that, then you should quit." Now that was a deal I could live with. For three sessions, I laid there. She looked so serious and busy as she sat quietly with her hands gently moving from place to place on my body. I felt nothing. By session four, I felt certain this well-intentioned lady was wasting her time with me. Although she assured me after each session I had several "good releases," I was pretty sure she was imagining anything she felt. I didn't want to call her a liar. I really enjoyed our time together. She was talking about emotional energy building up in our bodies, how sometimes we can let it build up to the point where there is no more room.

"Yes, the full cup, I could relate to that," I thought.

"So how do you empty your cup?" She talked about recognizing stressors and giving ourselves time and space to grieve, to cry, and to experience sadness and anger.

"Not suck it up?"

"No, definitely not. When you 'suck it up,' it can get stuck. Your body absorbs it, and if it's not allowed to be processed and released, a blockage forms."

I certainly felt "blocked." Wow, these were weird concepts; could any of this be accurate? If what she was saying was true, I had accumulated some serious, large blockages over the past year. If the Holy Spirit was like a river flowing through me, the river had some serious boulders in its path. In fact, it felt like there were probably a couple of big dams along the way, too. Where were the boulders? Were they causing more physical damage? Had they contributed to the cancer initially? Why does one's body turn against itself and form tumors that can destroy life? Maybe my suck-it-up mentality really wasn't healthy. Maybe the anxiety over cancer had been sucked up in there and was stuck now. I wanted it out. I needed to be flushed clean from anxiety and fear. I wanted to sleep normally, function normally. I wanted to be healthy and to stay healthy. I knew several breast cancer survivors and most seemed to deal with post-treatment emotional fallout with Prozac, Paxil, or Zoloft. I didn't want to take any more pills. I was disillusioned with the whole Western medicine mentality of poison, cut and burn; if it hurts, take a pill.

Maybe these Eastern concepts had more validity than I had been willing to admit. After all, they had been around for over 3000 years. There had to be some validity to them. I desired a natural cure, one that allowed my body and emotions to heal at their own rate. I knew God had created my body to be a miraculous healing machine. I remembered reading the chapter in Darwin's evolution book called "That Damned Eye," where Darwin vented his frustration regarding our amazing, self-healing eye, which defied all logic of evolution. The fact is that any minor trauma to the eye will heal within twenty-four hours. There is no way for science to explain these phenomena. A little known fact is that Darwin actually did not believe in evolution when he died, and a great deal of his unbelief came from studying the human body's capacity to heal itself. I wanted to tap into that God-given life stream of healing. I desperately desired emotional healing. I was tired of walking around with a full cup. I felt as though I was on the verge of tears most days. I was an emotional train wreck. Just as I had allowed the doctors at Stanford to use chemo to treat the cancer, I desperately needed to treat this flood of emotions that consumed me.

Toward the end of my fourth craniosacral session, I was thinking how much I would miss this fine lady. I hoped the Stanford clinic would be able to shed some light on my sleep problem. "Oh well, at least I gave this thing a shot." Lila moved to my left arm and extended it. I sighed and wondered how much time was left in our session. I glanced over to see my arm lazily trace a circle in the air. "Are you moving my arm?" Her touch was so light that I couldn't imagine how she could move my arm without my feeling any pressure.

"No, I'm just following the movement of your arm."

"My arm is moving itself?"

"Yes, it's called unwinding. It's perfectly natural." My arm felt detached from my body. I watched it move as a casual observer. "What's it unwinding from?"

"I don't know, it's obviously what your body needs right now. It's part of the body's process of healing itself."

Really. My body was healing itself. Now that was a concept I could latch onto. I didn't know how, why, or what my body was doing, but I knew I was going to come back and see what else my body needed.

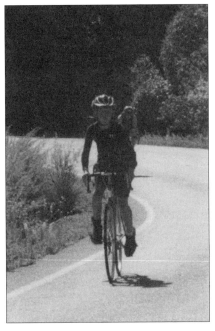

## 13

*Bryce in his first triathlon.*

# UVAS Triathlon

With two weeks remaining of my daily trek to Merced for radiation, our next triathlon loomed. I had registered for this tri the previous fall with hopes that it would be my all-my-treatment-is-done celebration. The extra surgery had set back my treatment schedule, so I had been training for all-my-treatment-is-*almost*-done triathlon. I had only been riding a couple times a week. A morning ride used all my energy for the day, so I spent those afternoons lying low. But emotionally, it was worth it. Being able to complete a ride was a huge emotional lift, and I couldn't give it up. In fact, the hardest ride we do, a cruise to the detention dam about fifteen miles from our home, was my post-chemo tradition. The third week post each chemo, when I felt as good as it would get, I rode my bike to the d-dam. There is a hill there that is a killer. It is total exhilaration to fly down, but you pay the price getting back up. I climbed this hill after each chemo; it was how I knew I was going to live. As long as I could endure that ride, I knew I would be OK. The last couple of weeks, I had been increasing the intensity of my swim workouts in anticipation of the looming tri.

When I was working out was the only time I felt I had any control over my body. It was the only way I knew to make myself stronger. During workouts, I felt like I was in control, instead of the cancer. The extreme fatigue that the workouts created was a tradeoff, but it was worth it.

With two weeks left until the tri, I decided it was the I-Beat-Cancer Tri. It still seemed beyond comprehension that I even had it, let alone beat it. The tri was to symbolize the end of sickness, end of tiredness, end of feeling like a poster child for breast cancer. I was actually proudly sporting an inch of hair! This tri would signal the end of the ever present "How are you feeling?" question from every encounter. Although I greatly appreciated everyone's concern, I longed not to be the object of their attention and concern.

The UVAS Reservoir is tucked into Hecker Pass, a beautiful mountain pass that dumps into the Pacific Ocean. The reservoir is surrounded by Eucalyptus trees and grape vineyards. Since this tri took place in May, the swim required a wetsuit. The water was definitely cold, but I love open water swims. I oddly feel surrounded and protected by large, murky waters. My son Bryce and two friends formed a team to join me. My friend Kathy swam; Bryce was on the bike, and Shelly had been training for the run. The swim was a blast; competition is just plain fun. I jumped onto my bike, and as Kathy tagged Bryce, we rode off along the beautiful tree-lined street that circled the reservoir. The scenery was gorgeous and peaceful. I was so thankful to be alive and healthy with enough energy to participate. Bryce had not figured out the gear thing. "I don't need to change it, Mom, I'll be fine."

But the course was gently rolling hills that cried out for rapid gear changes. Then came the killer climb. Bryce was already frustrated from riding the rolling hills in one gear, and the climb put him over the edge.

He jumped off and began to run with his bike up the long hill. He was fighting tears of frustration as I pulled over, "Here buddy, hold my bike for a minute." I jumped on his bike and rode downhill long enough to downshift, then rode back up to him and switched bikes. He took off and smiled over at me with an adorable look of sweaty relief. It was such a blessing to be riding along with my little buddy. When asked later what he felt when he found out I had cancer he said, "I was really scared, Mom. I thought you were going to die at first. Then after a couple of days, I thought it was kinda cool. I knew you were going to fight and win."

Today we were celebrating winning together. He looked so cute. At nine, he was the youngest competitor and less than half the size of most riders. I lagged behind and just enjoyed watching his little bottom with his little head tucked down in determination. Sixteen miles is a long way for a little body. But the end of the ride came too soon for me; it had been such a thrill. Now *The Run* loomed. Bryce tagged Shelly, and together we slogged it out. Neither one of us derives pleasure from running, but we were on a mission that day, and I was so thankful to have her beside me. We blazed through in eleven-minute miles. More importantly, we finished. As I crossed the finish line, I experienced a huge tightening pressure in my chest. I exhaled an excruciating grunt-wheeze I recognized as a huge release that Lila would be proud of—I was filled with emotion and my cup was ready to slosh. After the hugs, I escaped to a quiet spot and let it all out. I cried out of pure relief and thankfulness for my health. I had felt abandoned by my health, but now my health was restored. My journey through loss was long, and at the bottom, the only thing left was the love of God. But being alone with the love of God allowed me to discover the absolute fullness of life.

# 14

## Let the Healing Begin

---

I anticipated pure, free-flowing joy when my treatment was done. I was dead wrong. I had heard at the beginning of my treatment that post treatment could be the roughest part. Of course, I figured they were just lunatics. There's no way. Absolutely no way.

Well, it wasn't as bad as chemo, but it was certainly a very close second. My friends planned a Yahoo! It's Over Party at a local restaurant. I cancelled. I just wasn't in a celebrating mood, and it haunted me. The cancer is gone. Why don't I feel like celebrating? I cried, I moped, I was depressed. People would congratulate me, "Way to go, it's over!" but I would smile and pretend enthusiasm.

"What is wrong with me?" My support system dissipated, the nightmare was finally over for them, but I was a mess. At my next Stanford checkup, my intolerance for mutts reached its crescendo.

This particular resident was from some country on a European continent. I was guessing it was one of those countries liberated when the Berlin Wall came down. I could narrow it to a country where bathing and hair grooming were not a priority. This well-intentioned woman was determined to give me a thorough exam. After the usual litany of questions, she casually flipped through my thick chart. "I see you're scheduled to receive another few rounds of chemo."

I froze. "Not that I know of," I feigned casualness. This is just another nut that does not have a clue; nonetheless, I had been shaken to the core. Rick jumped in with questions, and she excused herself from the room. Rick and I held each other as we awaited Dr. Carmon's arrival. "I'm not scheduled for more chemo, right Honey?"

"No, she has no idea what she's talking about. Don't worry about it; don't even talk to her until Carmon gets here."

She brought her thick accent back into the room. "I'm sorry, Mrs. Howard, my mistake. You are done with your chemotherapy treatments."

Very huge sigh of relief.

"Now if you'll just lie back, I'll begin my exam."

Every cell in my body was screaming "No," but the old, "You gotta start somewhere, you've got to practice, right?" kept ringing in my head. This poor lady. Who knows what adversity she's gone through to get here? Her heavy, unsure hands were palpating my breast. She stopped, backed up, palpated again. Alarm bells immediately rang. What's going on?

"Is this lump the same size, or has it changed?"

My cup sloshed; my dam broke. First more chemo, now the cancer is back. The tears started rolling. I was sliding down the slope, gaining momentum toward no control at all-out sobbing. Rick came over and felt the offended area. "It's felt like this since surgery. It's exactly the same. We're going to wait for Dr. Carmon now. Thank you." I sat up and tried to compose myself as Eastern European Woman glared at us and exited the room.

A few minutes later, Dr Carmon came in to smooth things out. But by this time, I was a blubbering mess. I sat in the chair in the corner as Rick and Carmon talked. Rick explained what Eastern European Woman had said and done but all Carmon saw and heard was my crying. "Have you been emotional lately?" I nodded as I sniffed and wiped my swollen face. "I'm going to hook you up with a social worker. I think you'll find her very helpful." All I could think of was more trips to this hospital, a place I preferred to avoid at all costs.

She was actually very sweet and comforting. We sat in her cramped office with books stacked all around. "You know how when something happens to one of your kids, something really serious, and you hold it together to take care of the situation, and when the crisis is over you lay down and cry? It's the same thing you're experiencing now."

I nodded and sniffed and wiped as she talked. This made sense. "I'm going to set you up with a psychologist, and you can get some help." I continued to nod and sniff. We left with her business card and the promise of a follow-up call. She did call with an appointment, but I now had hope in Lila. I did not want to go to Stanford for anything other than what was absolutely necessary.

I decided to go to craniosacral therapy once a week. I didn't feel a lot happening, but I knew I felt better when I left—that is, until the sobbing began. But even that felt like a huge relief. I didn't know what I was crying about, but some force deep within me seemed to be pushing it out, and when I was done, I felt better. Lila explained it much as the psychologist had, "You have stuffed emotions down for a year. Be tough, suck it up . . . ignore your feelings and your fears. Just because you stuffed them down does not mean they went away. They were just shoved deeper. Now they're coming out."

As much as I hated crying, I just knew that it felt so good and cleansing to let it out. And if letting it out was going to help me sleep, then come on out, baby. I appreciated the quiet time in my car on the drive home. I couldn't believe it was possible to cry so much. I was embarrassed. I told no one of my new cleansing routine. But I started feeling better. My cup didn't feel full all the time. I remembered the shortest verse in the Bible: "Jesus wept."

"Lord, if you can cry, then so can I. It's OK to cry. What's not OK is holding it inside. I started studying the concept of weakness. "When you are weak, then I am strong." How does that work? Maybe He allows me to be weak, so He can be strong through me. He obviously wanted me weak, because He had so consistently held me in that place for a long time. Maybe when I was weak, I didn't get in the way of Him using me.

Cranial sessions became more intense and infinitely stranger. I was learning that God made our bodies considerably more complex than I ever imagined. This certainly was beyond anything I had learned in nursing school. My body had obviously stored every shred of emotional trauma I had felt but refused to acknowledge. Everything I had stuffed inside had made itself a cozy home in my body. And given the opportunity, my body was now looking to shed all the extra cargo it had accumulated. Our bodies want to heal. I learned that given the right environment, our bodies will heal themselves.

My cup was full when, in fact, God desires that our cups be empty. Empty, so he can totally flow through us. I had so many blockages that the Holy Spirit had to flow around that I could not effectively be used by Him. When blockages are removed, the Holy Spirit can flow openly, freely, and effectively. I was in the process of opening the flow.

The sessions intensified more than I ever thought possible. Aching, groaning, intense shooting pains. Lila would locate what she called the *energy cyst*, which, after time, I came to recognize as feeling like a small tornado swirling just beneath my skin. This tornado could be anywhere from dime size to the size of my abdomen and could be located anywhere on my body. I didn't fully understand how or why, I just knew that I really felt it. These tornadoes inevitably carried with them the next layer of emotion my body was ready to release, and I never knew what emotion was about to burst out. Most sessions were just plain unpleasant. Where did all this come from? Was it all cancer related? The process of craniosacral therapy caused extreme thirst, and I drank water constantly. Lila said my body was flushing. I sure hoped so.

Was not sleeping the result of craniosacral therapy? No. Was not sleeping God's way of keeping me going to craniosacral therapy? Yes. I was feeling more convicted and peaceful that it's from God. Lila is a gift from God. With one hand, He's allowing me to experience insomnia; with the other hand He's leading me to thorough healing and understanding, while keeping me motivated to continue moving toward healing.

I badly wanted Rick to experience this. "Lord, if you want me in it, I know you'll work it out so Rick will come on board and experience and understand. I can't take this road without him." I would not have stayed in the room with that uncomfortable experience if I had not been highly motivated.

# 15

## Insomnia

Insomnia now dominated my life. I was ashamed of my complete dependence on sleeping pills. Some nights I took up to five or six sleeping pills before finally passing out. I tried different combinations of anti-anxiety drugs and sleeping pills. I read until all hours. I plowed through more books than I've ever read in my life. Usually I took one pill and waited an hour before taking the next pill. Four or five hours later, the anger and frustration peaked, putting sleep even further out of my reach. Rolling over, I'd flick my bedside light on and with burning, bleary eyes force myself to read for another hour before allowing myself another opportunity for sleep. When morning arrived, I groggily opened my eyes, thankful that another miserable night had passed and wondering how many more I would have to endure this way. I was miserable.

By now, I had cleaned out the shelf at our local health food store. Any supplement or tea that promised sleep, I tried. Yoga, meditation, headphones with softly playing music, pleasantly scented eye patches that promised relaxation and guaranteed sleep. I even spent some time at an oxygen bar. None of it worked. My weekly cranial sessions continued.

The next week during cranial, I felt overwhelming sadness and frustration. I understood I felt vulnerable and weak during cancer, two feelings I despised. Now I understood vulnerable and weak could be a good thing. God uses us in our weakness; and when we are vulnerable and open, He can more efficiently work through us. Our basic nature is weak, and that's OK.

The following week I settled in on the now familiar table. Although the sessions were consistently unpleasant, I knew I was making positive progress and looked forward to my trips to this place of healing. With Lila's hands gently on my body, it didn't take long until I felt a knot in my abdomen and severe burning in my left breast. It became difficult to breathe; I felt the knot extending to my battered breast. What the heck is this? My right breast felt like there were twenty bungee cords connecting it to my womb. It felt secure. My left breast, the cancer breast, felt floating, unattached, insecure. I had the overwhelming desire to connect my weak breast to my womb again. I prayed for wisdom, "Whatever Lord, I do not understand; but please help me."

I began the connection process. Crying, stretching-bungee mentally from my womb to my left breast, stretch . . . stretch . . . strain . . . ah, connected now, connected . . . to my weak self. Ah, it is so weird, but it feels so right. Yes, I am weak, but it's OK now. I've always been weak. I just didn't want to admit it. I only tried to act strong. Only by God's grace am I allowed any strength. My basic nature is weak, and that's OK. Now I'm weak and whole. Most importantly, now He can use me more efficiently.

Reliving the emotional aspects of chemo was excruciating. The first ugly flashback began innocently with a feeling of widening in my chest, as if someone was performing open-heart surgery on me. My chest cavity was slowly being cranked open, inch by excruciating inch. The pain slowly intensified. I started crying and kept thinking, "I let them poison me! My body is Christ's temple, and I let them poison me!" I remembered how it took eight sticks to start the IV after chemo number three. My body had shut down and wasn't going to let them in. Now I understood.

Lila standing with her hands lightly on my chest . . . I could feel the tornado growing and yelled out. "I hate Carmon!" I hated him for telling me I was tolerating the chemo well and continuing to poison me even after I was so obviously sick. I said I hated all the nurses who poisoned me too. I know chemo had to happen. It saved my life, but I absolutely hated the process.

After that exhausting session, I came home and went for a long run. At the end of the run, crying, I lifted my hands in the air. I gave chemo, Carmon, and cancer to God. I pushed it up with my hands and my breath and sensed a cocoon of cotton surrounding all three. The cocoon was attached to a string that God pulled, taking it all to heaven. "It's all yours, Lord. Thank you for letting me experience this and letting me grow."

I felt anger, fear, resentment, abandonment; they all were all broiling around inside me. I desperately wanted it all out, every last drop of it. But it felt like I had a brick wall to break through. Can I ever break down this wall? Each brick was some emotion I had "sucked up," and the bricks were stacked high and deep. Could I ever really recognize and process each emotion I had so unwittingly stacked on this wall? I understood now how and why so many people spend their entire lives hiding behind their brick wall. It's safe there. The wall is protection. My heart ached as I thought of people with years of trauma, years of building walls and hiding just to survive.

I knew I didn't want to live my life hunkered down behind this wall. Now that I knew it was there and what it was composed of, I was determined to break it down. Like the Berlin Wall crashing down, I knew freedom was on the other side, freedom from emotional trauma, freedom from anti-anxiety pills, freedom from incessant hyperventilating, and freedom from insomnia. I was determined to let all of the emotions out, layer by painful layer.

I did a lot of praying, "Lord, I really do believe you are who you say you are, that you love me, but where were you the last ten months? I know you were letting me go through this so I could be stronger, but a portion of me still says, "Where were you? I felt you allowing suffering with one hand and holding and comforting me with the other. Faithfulness. You are faithful; but deep down, I still feel the ache of abandonment and anger. I know that's the ache that's constantly in my chest. Lila says it's a privilege to wrestle with God at this point in my life, instead of on my deathbed like most people. I did feel this wrestling with God in the beginning, when I questioned why He was allowing me to go through this. But I just had to grit my teeth and go. Now I need to resolve this, be done with it. I really feel I need to not go at it so hard for a while, need to relax and just let God love me for now.

I took a few weeks off. I needed to rest and stop fighting and thinking, to allow God to heal all the rawness that had been exposed. A month later, I was back at it.

"Cranial was so intense this week. It was so phenomenally weird. If people knew about this stuff, I'm afraid they'd lock me up. But these emotions are in my body, uncomfortably roiling around. And it feels so good to let it out. Pain in my right breast. Intense pain. Now when I feel pain in an area, I ask my body what it is. "What emotional trauma is stored there?" Usually I get the answer. The answer comes like a billboard lighting up in my mind. It's so weird. I asked what the breast pain was and instantly I knew it was anger. Anger at Dr Denis, anger at his passive, cool, calculating dissertation regarding the odds of survival on *my* life. Anger at the hospital for withholding my pain meds, anger for throwing up twelve hours post surgery because the nurse didn't give me my Zofran shot, anger at the anesthesiologist for giving me the wrong sedative, which caused the puking, anger at Rick for not protecting me from all this trauma, even though there's nothing he could have done . . ." So much anger coming out. I was still a mess, still not sleeping, but I knew I was making progress.

Subsequent cranials unearthed old high school injuries. That felt highly unproductive, but I knew I had to get through that layer to get to what was underneath. Maybe the next layer would help with my sleep, but no, the next layer dealt with the menopause chemotherapy had induced. Lila, with her hands lightly on my abdomen, my stomach felt like it was swirling. "Menopause," I whispered incredulously. The billboard sign had flashed in my mind. This process continued to mystify and amaze me. "How long did it take for menopause to occur with you?"

"Well, one month after chemo started. My period stopped."

"How long does menopause normally take?" She obviously knew the answer but always waited for me to figure things out on my own. It was part of the process.

"Years."

"Well, it feels like your body is working out the details of that sudden cessation."

I came home and practiced feeling Rick's rhythm. He fell asleep in ten minutes. The dear man was enduring my visits with Lila, but obviously I hesitated even sharing with him what happened when I was in that room. It was all so weird. At the same time, I wanted him to understand that I was making progress and to understand the process I was going through. I got my share of eye rolls when we sat down for the *let me tell you what happened at cranial today* talk. Through it all, he was kind and supportive and did his best to understand.

I finally felt I had moved past the anger and abandonment feelings. Sleep was slightly improved. I was able to establish a rhythm of one pill one hour before sleep, reading, and blissfully falling asleep for eight hours. I still could rarely fall asleep for naps. When I was blessed with a short nap, I had an amazing, energy-filled afternoon. Those days gave me a glimpse of *normal*. I started working out less to conserve energy.

The next session was deep and disturbing. I had lots of abdominal cramping and then thoughts of cancer, visions of gooey black tar in my left breast. Satan wants cancer and fear to be my weakness. It's his way of controlling me, but I won't give in. God is in control. Lots of time in prayer. I finally understood that it's a spiritual battle. Because all of life, ultimately, is a spiritual battle.

It was summer vacation. I had two months before I was scheduled to return to work. "I am so blessed to have this down time from work for recovery, revival, and refreshing . . ."

I struggle with responsibilities. What really is *my* responsibility and what is God's? I need to learn to not carry concerns, fears, and worries regarding other people. We're not meant to carry the load. God is. We do what we feel led to do and give the rest to Him. Carrying the load is unhealthy and unproductive. I am imperfect, just like God made me. I need to rest in God's mercy and grace. It is sufficient for me. He died so that I could have mercy and grace abundantly. As a parent is pleased with a child's performance but doesn't demand perfection, so God is pleased with us. He still loves us totally, just as a parent loves their child.

I had dreamed constantly of Hawaii during treatment. "When I finish treatment, I am going to Hawaii. I am going to sit in the sun, swim in the ocean, and just do whatever I want!" I dreamed of the warm ocean during chemo. I dreamed of it during all those hours on the couch. But when the time finally arrived, Rick balked. "Hawaii is just too hot and muggy in the summer. We can do Hawaii this winter. How about an Alaskan cruise this summer?"

I had the Harriet syndrome. I feared healing for a short time and then, "Oops! Now it's in your lungs." Would I still be healthy by winter? I explained my fears to Rick.

"It's over, Honey; it's never coming back." He held me tightly. "We'll do both vacations." Was he in denial again? It's never coming back? How could he be so confident? And how could I be so consumed with fear and doubt?

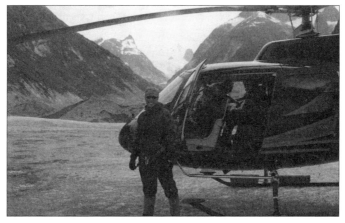

## 16

*My amazing glacier hike in Alaska.*

# Alaska

Alaska is simply spectacular. During my college days, my girl-friend Terry and I worked one summer in Dillingham, Alaska, at a salmon processing plant. We worked for a couple of months, and then hitchhiked around the interior of Alaska before flying to Hawaii to spend the last few dollars we had earned. We had an awesome time, and I was anxious to see more of this beautiful state.

The ports we now visited had definitely adapted to the cruise-ship industry. No longer were they rustic little towns. Now they reminded me of Disneyland or, worse, Hollywood. The ports were all dressed up and phony, a thousand shops all selling the same trinkets. They reminded me of the fake movie sets we had seen at Universal Studios in Los Angeles. I expected to look behind them and see bare cardboard. "This is not Alaska! The real Alaska is in there," I pointed, "beyond all that glitz and show."

What had they done with this gorgeous wilderness state? At the first port, I insisted we hike. We had to get past all the storefronts, so I could show Rick the Alaska I remembered. Unfortunately, the port was at the bottom of a hill, and the "real deal" was exasperatingly uphill. Walking around the pasture to check his cows was Rick's idea of exercise. He had had his fill of workouts in football.

"I'm not walking all the way up this hill, Honey. Let's just go back."

"No! You've got to see how pretty it is!" I knew there was a park at the top of this hill, so close, and yet so far. A garbage truck rumbled toward us, and my old Alaska instincts took over. I stuck my thumb out, and he obligingly pulled over.

"What are you doing? I'm not riding in that thing!" I flashed him a grin as I grabbed the rung to pull myself up to the door.

"Come on, Babe. This is gonna be fun!" The garbage man was predictably friendly and accommodating. It was the Alaskan way. We chatted as the old stinky truck whined up the steep hill. When he pointed out the trailhead, we hopped out and waved goodbye. The hike was gorgeous. Within minutes, it felt like we were in the middle of a dense forest. It smelled so good; the undergrowth was lush and green. Water dripped from the trees to the moss and fern below. "Now this is Alaska, Honey. Isn't it wonderful?"

He was a trooper. We arrived at the end of the trail, which offered a lookout point with spectacular views. We could clearly see our cruise ship in the port far below with a steady stream of people boarding. We ran, hopped, and skidded back down the trail, out past the dump, and down to the port. We had glimpsed the real Alaska!

My husband was in a magnanimous mood. "Take whatever excursions you want, Babe." He pointed out the mountain biking trip outlined in our cruise brochure. Rick considered any bike seat to be a health hazard. I would be on my own. There was also a helicopter flight to a glacier listed, and the brochure mentioned hiking around the glacier with crampons. Oh, yeah, definitely something I need to try, but a 250-pound maximum weight was listed for helicopter passengers. I would be on my own. A kayaking excursion looked like something we would both enjoy. We ordered up our fun for the week.

It was so relaxing being away with Rick, but I still didn't feel right. So many anxieties were still frustratingly broiling around inside. I had hoped when I got away from home that all of my anxieties and fears would somehow disappear, maybe stay behind in Los Banos and give me a break. It just wasn't to be. Even surrounded by the beauty and fun of Alaska, my insomnia continued. I now understood that I couldn't run far enough to get away from it. It was a part of me. "I haven't felt *right* for so long. I don't know if I'll even recognize it. When will this all be resolved?"

## 17

# Healing Continues

$B$ack at home, I was incredulous at the waves of anger toward God that I was still experiencing. There were several uncomfortable days with uncontrollable waves of crying. "Just go with it," I kept telling myself. "Let it out." Swimming was a wonderful outlet, and one afternoon, I swam about fifty laps of butterfly while crying. I swam as fast and as hard as I could, but I still wasn't tired. Normally five or six laps did me in. I hoped that I had burned up some of that anger.

"I'm mad that I got cancer! I'm mad that you allowed me to get Cancer! Why did you let this happen to me?"

"It's a process, a journey, to get where you need to be," came the soft, reassuring voice from somewhere deep inside my head.

"Will I live to see my kids grow up?"

I asked for a trip to Aptos, alone. It was a once in a lifetime experience. Just me and my bike. I slept in, read in bed and drank coffee, (one of my favorite luxuries), kept a journal, and prayed. "Teach me, Lord. Pour your wisdom and desires into me, I'm open."

I took off one afternoon and rode to Santa Cruz, up and around those beautiful mountains. It was so awesome and peaceful. I had not been alone like that since college. I felt guilty asking Rick after he'd already done so much, but he is so wonderful and supportive. I was feeling the overwhelming desire to be alone to heal and pray. I had three days.

Like the waves, a little at a time . . . life is a process, never one big tidal wave but a steady, slow process. *In due time* . . . I will heal and find peace *in due time* . . . patience.

I had a dream last night that Rick and I were driving around a steep mountain curve and went off the edge. I was praying all the way down, "Lord, please protect the kids, please be with us." We woke up on our couches with no cuts or bruises—totally fine! Maybe this means the cancer is not coming back and that I can live free. It was a journey to give me wisdom and more understanding tuned into the Holy Spirit. Was it worth it? Yes!

I signed up for the Craniosacral Therapy I (CST) class offered in San Francisco. I couldn't wait to learn just how this amazing process works. I was shocked and impressed at the number and variety of classes offered. Rick made fun of me. He told me to be sure and take a tie dye shirt so I would fit in with the crowd.

It was a phenomenal four days. I was very impressed with the caliber of people enrolled in my class. An MD, nurses, physical therapists, chiropractors, dentists, massage therapists. The entire scope of healthcare providers was represented. And, yes, there were a couple of tie-dye, Birkenstock-wearing, granola-eating folks in the room, but the rest of the crowd was all people just like me! I looked around the room and wondered what had brought these people to this place? What was their story? Had everyone, or anyone, had a dramatic experience with CST like I had? Had they just stumbled onto this class as a means of fulfilling their professional continuing education requirements?

I was sitting next to a chiropractor, so I asked her why she was at the class. "Sue" had learned the CST soft-tissue release techniques from a chiropractor in her office. She had used them successfully with her patients and was anxious to expand her understanding of soft-tissue releases. I met a physical therapist who now used CST techniques exclusively in her practice. She had become disillusioned with the old ice pack and weights rehab routine. After she started using CST soft-tissue releases she began experiencing huge success. Her practice was packed, and her business was booming with satisfied patients. I spoke with an ObGyn who was incorporating CST into his practice. He was excited about CST, and he is gathering data regarding the significantly decreased demand for medication during childbirth when CST is incorporated into the labor process.

I learned that the craniosacral system consists of the membranes and cerebrospinal fluid that surrounds the brain and spinal cord. Thus the name cranial, from the cranium of the skull down to the sacrum or sacral. Since all of our nerves originate from the spinal cord and travel the entire length of our bodies, the craniosacral rhythm can be felt anywhere. Ah! The lights were going on. Now I understood how Lila could stand at my feet and feel the *rhythm* she always talked about . . . the light-touch techniques that were used enable therapists to treat the source of the problem rather than the symptoms. Ah! The source would be the *tornadoes* I felt, or *energy cysts* as Lila referred to them. I learned that the fascia system in our body is like a *superman suit* pulled on just under our skin.

When energy enters the body, from either a physical or emotional trauma, it can get stuck if the body or mind does not process it. (Yes, that would be the old "suck it up" or "ignore it and it will go away" method so many of us use.) The resulting excess energy compacts itself to cause as little harm as possible to the body. That energy can then swirl around indefinitely. The resulting tornado causes restrictions, or interruptions, to the fascia system. Think of a shirt pulled down with two fingers along the bottom edge. The effects of that tug can clearly be seen up on the shoulder. Try it! You'll see the wrinkles extending up to affect almost every inch of the fabric. Our body logically works the same way. A restriction in the fascia near the foot, or the source, can actually cause pain in the shoulder, the symptom. Wow. This was making sense. It was such a relief to have everything I had experienced emotionally and physically in the last six months confirmed physiologically and scientifically. After all, energy is all around us. The basic building blocks of our cells, the protons and electrons, maintain their integrity and structure by energetically opposing each other. Without energy, our bodies would literally collapse. Why was it so difficult to conceptualize that we could, when trained, actually feel this energy? And now I knew what it felt like. I was transfixed by this whole process.

I knew that the deep emotional trauma I had unwittingly sucked up had formed who knows how many of those ugly tornadoes, which were now packed away in my body in layers. As each tornado was energetically released, I experienced the flood of emotions that tornado contained. It all made sense.

We practiced feeling each other's craniosacral rhythm. The CS rhythm is separate and distinct from breathing and heart rate. The flow of the cerebrospinal fluid around the spinal column resembles a semi-enclosed hydraulic chamber, and this system creates a predictable and distinct ebb and flow rhythm. There it was! I was definitely feeling it! Like tuning into a hard to find radio station, one more slight turn of the knob and sudden clarity. There it was, loud and clear! I was loving this stuff. Having felt my body respond to the gentle manipulations Lila used had been amazing, but actually facilitating the releases on someone else was just plain phenomenal! I was totally, awed, amazed, and deeply moved by this whole energy dimension of life that God created and I had been unaware of.

And how could it be that something so powerful, so healing, could be such a secret, a relative unknown in the medical field? Why had I never heard of this? Subsequent readings revealed the answer to my provocative question. Simply, there is no money to be made in this field. There are no drugs to be sold, no machines to peddle. Solid, dynamic research that proves the efficiency of energetic healing routinely is quietly shelved. Who's going to make money off this stuff? Research journals are all funded by drug companies. They won't publish these research results.

Surging with the energy I could now actually feel, I came home to five bodies. I was going to do a lot of practicing on these five beautiful bodies. Rick's heel was really bothering him. I had been giving him nightly foot massages. Now I added CST. I felt lots of shifting going on inside, but he felt nothing. *In due time.*

Our annual triathlon at New Melones was approaching fast. I was disappointed to admit I was in worse shape than during the previous year, when I had been in the middle of chemotherapy. I had been unable to run at all for the last six months. My hands and feet were still numb and uncomfortable, the last lingering side effect from chemotherapy. They constantly bothered me. I was confident about the bike and swim portions; the run would just have to work itself out.

The swim was as exhilarating as always. Despite some mild body bumping, we cruised the distance easily. We ran up the dock, hopped on our bikes, and then the real fun began. The sixteen-mile course consisted of rolling hills, my favorite, and it was a blast. All too soon, it was time for the run. The cross-country course consists of two, two-mile laps. As I slogged through the first lap, I chatted with myself regarding the possibility of completing one lap and heading home. "Don't be a quitter," was the voice on the right side of my head. "Who are you trying to impress, anyway? Just do what you can comfortably do, and head in!" was the dissenting voice from the left. They started duking it out.

"Quit!" "Finish!" "Quit" "Finish!" As I neared the fork in the path, the skirmish increased in intensity. "Who cares? Your feet hurt. Just head in, you bonehead!" "Don't you dare quit, you'll be a quitter! You hate quitters!" The left side apparently won, as I was dismayed and yet equally relieved to see I was headed home. As I crossed the finish line, I glanced up at the electronic timer to see that I had finished, or almost finished, in the same time it took me to do the entire tri last year. Oh well, at least I was done. I walked back to find Rick and told him what I had done.

"It's alright, Honey, it doesn't matter! You did great!" As some faster runners finished behind me, I found myself explaining to more people than I desired that I had cut my run short. I was embarrassed.

The post-race barbecue is held in a quaint park in Angel's Camp. There are always lots of good food and ice cold drinks. As we downed our lunch, an announcer began handing out the age group award winners. I froze and glanced over at Rick, "You don't suppose . . .?"

He shrugged his shoulders, shook his head, "Nah, don't worry about it."

"And with second place in the women's forty- to forty-five-year-old division, Sandy Howard!"

I jerked straight up, eyes wide. "Oh no! I didn't earn that! I'm cheating the rightful winner." My mind raced. Do I explain to the officials how I had cheated? Oh, why did I ever cross that finish line? I should have just stopped short so my time wouldn't have been officially recorded. I had not even thought about this scenario during my Rocky session.

Rick's voice cut in on my thoughts, "Babe, just go get the medal."

"But . . ."

"Just walk up there and get it." After a lot of much-deserved razzing, I came home and put the undeserved metal face down in the back of a drawer.

I made the appointment and sat back with satisfaction. The time had finally arrived. I heaved a deep sigh and tears welled in my eyes. It was finally over; this was really going to happen. *In due time*…the time was finally due…. for my first haircut. The frizzy ends were trimmed off, some gel was applied. She swirled it around and tried to make the moment last. I cried tears of relief.

And then, finally, the ultimate cranial session, the moment I had been praying for: Lila, with her hands on my diaphragm, rippling, cramping. "Go down there with your mind and see if you can tell what this is."

Billboard: "Fear!" I just knew it.

"What does it look like?"

"A huge cloud."

"How big is the cloud?"

"The size of Texas."

"What are you going to do with it?"

I prayed for the answer and finally visualized a huge, heavenly vacuum. I prayed for God to take all the fear, and soon it felt like the vacuum was sucking the cloud heavenward. This process took a very long time. It was totally exhausting work. I finally thought I was done, when I realized the cloud of fear was also completely underneath me. I initially thought the cloud was just on top of me, but now I could see it had surrounded me. "Agh! Too much! Don't stop! Keep going!"

Lila suggested that I could save part of the work and finish next week.

No way. I was exhausted, but I had to finish. Now that I had seen this mass of fear, there was no way I was carrying it one step further. After more exhausting vacuuming, the cloud was gone. But like a huge abalone anchored on, I could feel the last painful piece stuck to my left rib cage. Finally, with a huge pop and excruciating pain, the last piece was sucked up to heaven. God would carry the load for me now. I prayed and filled the empty space with God's divine and holy light. Lots of deep breaths later, dare I even think it? Was that it? Will I sleep tonight?

I am sleeping! I have slept four nights without pills! Yeah, I'm pretty stoked. Very stoked and very thankful. It was fear that kept me awake at night. Fear of dying a slow and painful death from cancer. I knew that was a huge fear of mine, and I felt I had given it to God. Obviously, subconsciously, I was holding onto that fear, and it had absolutely dominated my life.

I interestingly realized several days later that the exact spot where the fear was anchored had been the same place that had been painful throughout my pregnancy with Bryce. I was very anxious to have four healthy kids, and I guess I figured with three healthy kids already, the odds were increased that something could be wrong with Bryce. I walked around the entire pregnancy with my left hand jammed under my left rib cage. Putting pressure on the spot helped to ease the pain. Now I know that the pain had been fear.

I have been quarantined for five days. During my last three-month check up with Carmon, I showed them the pustules that had started itching that morning. "Look at these things! They're itchy and they look like chicken pox!"

A quick glance by Carmon confirmed my diagnosis.

"How can I get chicken pox? I've already had them!"

"It's not uncommon for post-chemo patients to get chickenpox. Your immune system has been compromised. Sometimes a dormant virus pops out. This can be very dangerous for you, though. I'd like to put you in the hospital for a couple days."

I cringed. I felt fine. "No thank you. I'll go home and rest. I'll be fine. No hospital."

Thankfully, he didn't push the issue, and I came home to quarantine myself. I had just been back at work for a month. I called my schools and explained the situation; I would be staying home for a week. They also took an aspiration from my lumpectomy site—Carmon didn't like the way it looked or felt—but it had looked the same since radiation ended. I called the next day and learned the pathology report was negative. I was relieved, but I hadn't been desperately worried. I am totally surrendered to God's will. Now Dr. Denis wants a core biopsy done. That fun is scheduled for the 18th. But I'm still not worried. And sleeping is great! Twelve-hour nights with this virus. Rest is a beautiful gift.

I started feeling very bad one day during my quarantine, tired, sad, no energy. I went and rested on my bed in the afternoon, but my body felt like it weighed 1,000 pounds. I remember thinking, "It's a good thing that I don't have to go to the bathroom, because if I did, I would just have to lay here and wet the bed." I truly felt that I could not move. Rick came in to ask me a question but I could not speak. He got irritated and left, but I didn't even care. He is under major stress right now with business, and I felt so guilty that I couldn't function. I would have panicked, but I knew I had cranial next morning. "Just be calm, ride the wave until I see Lila tomorrow."

It took all of my effort to get out of bed and get the kids off to school. I kept my head down so nobody would notice me or talk to me this morning. "Not feeling very well today, have a good day." They're so used to seeing mom at half speed, now they barely notice. Finally, quiet; just have to get to the car. Slumped over, "Please protect me from a wreck this morning, Lord." Cars are flying by me; how can people go so fast? Life is swarming around me, suffocating. I tell myself to make an effort to stand erect, to not draw any attention to myself as I walk straight back to *my room* where I slump in a chair to a wave of relief. "I know she will help me."

"Something's wrong…feel like someone… pulled the plug…I drained out… please help me," I whisper when Lila arrives.

It's such a relief to finally be on the table . . . Lila's gentle, reassuring touch and her confident, soft voice.

"Sometimes it's good to start over. This is an opportunity to take the pieces you like, keep them, and rebuild. Ask God to help you in this process; take your time. Pray, 'Where do I start? Lord, please help me find me, make me the person you want me to be.' "

Sorting through me, the parts I like, don't like, it's a laundry pile. Whites in this pile, darks over there. I feel like I'm slowly being knitted back together . . . I feel too weak to talk. "Don't panic, she will help me."

I walked in like a scarf unraveled; I walk out half a scarf with several dropped stitches. At home I go straight to bed. I will be fine. "Ride the wave. Lord, help me be whole again, please." I stay in bed for two days.

"Mom has the flu." The third day I'm feeling some energy; I'm coming back. What was that? I've never felt depression like that . . . a little PMS maybe. How do people live like that?

The biopsy went smoothly. I felt energetic and enthusiastic yesterday for the first time in six weeks. I have had cold, flu, chicken pox, depression. I go to work, come home, and sleep. Then yesterday, energy! "Thank you, Lord!" Now I understand that even though I'm sleeping, my stress will still be expressed in different ways. Somehow the layer that just came out caused my body to react by shutting down, depression style. I never got the "billboard" to understand what my body was releasing in that layer. I just hope I never have to feel that again. I have felt distance from God during illnesses. David, the author of the book of Psalms, and "a man after God's heart," frequently complained of God's apparent absence. David learned that God is more concerned that you trust Him than that you feel Him. "I will never leave you or forsake you." - Hebrews 13:5. I'm still learning the lesson of trust.

Happy New Year! It is a blessed, happy new year of health and healing and praise. I pray for continued growth and appreciation and love for others this new year. I pray for abounding, unselfish love. To love others with Christ's love, so they can understand a bit of Him through me— what an honor that would be—to balance caring for myself, listening to my body, and reaching out to others. To be aware of the Holy Spirit continuously through the day, always checking in, continual conversation, prayer. I am amazed at what a struggle it is to stay in touch spiritually, a daily struggle just to stay near the track—not even on it. But I have reached the outermost edges of understanding that it's not about me. This is just a trial run of all the awesomeness of eternity. I want to get it right.

I did cranial on Rick last night—did foot for a while and then head. Head was throbbing, which he actually felt. Lots of energy drained from his head. He could really feel the rhythm though he just barely acknowledged it. Can't wait to do it again. CST II class is next week. I can't wait to learn more.

CST II continues to fascinate. Totally mind-blowing. Phenomenal. More adjectives are redundant, but never would have I believed that I could feel such amazing things and sense so much information: Gently blend, ask permission, hold space, less is better. Unbelievable concepts that just plain work. So many times this weekend I have wished that I was a physical therapist so I could totally incorporate cranial into my practice—at the same time knowing God has me right where he wants me—not knowing where the cranial is taking me and at the same time at perfect peace.

Just as the Holy Spirit guides in cranial to amazing understanding, so he guides us in our life decisions and direction. The pull is equally strong. Please pull me, give me sensitivity, wisdom, understanding. Checkup last Thursday at Stanford. I was anxious; I couldn't fall asleep and had to take a pill. Next morning while praying, I heard Him say, "Be still, my child." Then I felt total peace. I went to the appointment with peace, and it's the first time we've been in and out with no surprises. For the first time I feel like I'm done with it. Totally done, a pretty awesome feeling.

What God does in us while we wait is as important as what we are waiting for.

Check-in was far too slow; the ocean was calling me. We grabbed our suits out of our bags, found a bathroom in the lobby, and dove into the beautiful, warm, Hawaiian water. "I'm here. I'm finally here." I had anticipated a complete melting away of all anxieties and concerns as soon as I sank into the warm, crystal-clear water. Like Alaska, it didn't happen. I mentally filed this disappointment away. I wouldn't let this ruin this spectacular trip.

We rented snorkel gear and searched out all the great spots. I absolutely adore spying on schools of fish as they dart from one area to the next. What are they looking for? Do they think? Feel? We watched schools of colorful fish for hours. Rick and I slowly glided along on the surface, heads submerged, holding hands, pointing out particularly colorful or energetic fish. "This is such a beautiful world you created, Lord. Thank you for this time to enjoy it." Back in our room, I burst into tears. I was thoroughly disgusted with myself. "Here you are in Paradise, and you still can't pull it together."

Rick came out of the shower to find me sniffling. "What's going on, Hon?"

"I still feel this anxiousness, this tightness in my chest. I hate this feeling. I thought maybe while I was here, it would decrease, or even go away. But it's still here."

Lots of hugs and encouragement later, I felt better. Not healed, but better. In years past, I would not have shared this with Rick. I would have stomped it down and said, "Suck it up!" and moved on. I was learning to let it out, to express my feelings completely, to be totally honest, and to move toward healing. This venting session served to deepen our relaxation and contentment for the remaining days of the trip. Rick really understood my turmoil. I found that sharing everything with him was a huge relief for me. He was so eager to help and support.

The trip over to the island of Lanai was a total blessing. We took a Kodiak around to the back of the island and found dolphins—oh, man— too exciting. I was screaming and hanging off the front of the Kodiak. We were in the middle of 100 or so dolphins. They were cruising right off our bow. I could have touched them if my arms were longer! I wanted to jump in so badly but was discouraged by talk of sharks in the area.

And on the way back to Maui, we saw whales breaching. Breathtaking. I cried when I saw the first one. As we sailed through *whale alley,* they became second nature. We saw so many somehow propel their enormous bodies straight out of the water. The sight was glorious. A mom and her baby put on a show for us. The baby breached at least four times, and it was spectacular! And so close! Almost too much for my poor heart.

I had a new development. I found a lump last week. Sheer terror and depression for three days. I finally gave it to God, so now I'm at peace during the day. I can function normally, but at night I can't sleep again. Trying to put all fear and anxiety in Jesus' hands but can't seem to get it all unloaded—back to sleeping pills. So frustrating. Want this desperately to be a false alarm but feel otherwise. "Not my will, but yours be done!" And that is tough. Putting my eye on the prize and not our present and minor afflictions.

On the outside it looks like things are falling apart on us. On the inside, where God is making new life, not a day goes by without His unfolding grace. These hard times are small potatoes compared to the coming times, the lavish celebration prepared for us. II Corinthians 4.

All is well. Ultrasound showed the lump to be scar tissue. A radiation boost causes tissue changes for up to three years. Wow. I felt like I had been in a refrigerator box with about three inches of space in front of my face. And as soon as I found out I was OK, the sides unzipped and my world opened back up. I could think about others' needs; I had energy for compassion and concern. I thought of people with so much to protect and hide, with their sides zipped up constantly, with no extra energy to reach out to others. I would hate to live my life that way.

And yet another testament to the effectiveness of craniosacral therapy: Three days before the lump appointment, my back cramped up and I could hardly walk. The next day, I made an appointment with Lila. My back was cramping continuously. I understand now that the cramping was my fear of cancer returning. I felt much better when I left Lila's; at least I could walk, despite a lot of discomfort. As soon as the ultrasound radiologist said the lump was normal tissue, I jumped off the table. My back pain disappeared. Unbelievable. I am continually amazed at how our tissue shuffles emotions around.

Rick's reaction to craniosacral therapy is so frustrating. I need to talk about my experiences with cranial and not worry about him rolling his eyes. Cranial yesterday was disgusting. Absolutely sickening. I'm still trying to sort it out. I had dry heaves within one minute of starting. My stomach was not nauseated like it had been in past cranials; I never felt like anything came up, just dry heaving—what was that?

We had a wonderful Fourth of July in Aptos—it was fun and relaxing with the Eriksons. We went to the beach, felt so good to feel cool air. Rick was relaxed; he napped and read. So good to see him relax. I have been doing weekly massages to help de-stress him. Each massage ends with fifteen minutes of cranial. I know it will help him eventually. *In due time. . .*

We finally sold the trailer park, which has created a tremendous change in his personality. He is understandably calmer now that he doesn't have to work twelve hours a day, seven days a week. We were so used to him being stressed out that we didn't really notice anymore. It just became a way of life. I can't believe how easy it was to slide toward perpetual fast forward. Each day was a race to see if he could get everything done. And now that one huge headache is gone, we can see the remarkable difference less stress makes in our lives. We are planning to sell one property a year until his life becomes balanced.

We throw open our doors to God and discover at the same moment that he has already thrown his door open to us. We find ourselves standing where we always hoped we'd stand, out in the wide-open spaces of God's grace and glory, standing tall and shouting praise. - Romans 5

Oh boy...very weird cranial yesterday. I had the overwhelming desire to lie on my stomach with my legs pulled up toward my head. My back arched, my head extended back toward my feet. Then my arms grabbed my legs. There I lay, looking like I had been hog-tied. So weird— no idea. Sore and exhausted today. Also very cranky. Not sleeping again for four nights. Think it's anxiety about the September 9 Stanford checkup. Trying, praying to be calm—very frustrating. Very tired.

The weirdness never stops. Next session, shoulders and neck twisting, circling around and around for an hour. Yeah, that's right, an hour. Next day, awesome swim. Amazing swim. Shoulders loose, I feel like I have the shoulders of a ten-year-old. You know how you hold a rubber band with one hand and wind it up? Just keep winding until the whole thing is tight and spiraled? Now picture letting go of one end. That's how my shoulders feel. Totally unwound. From what, I'll never know for sure, but I just can't help but think that whatever was there would have created arthritis or some other painful condition later in life.

Then, the last time was the right arm bending back as far behind me as possible, whipping in close in front. Repeated this motion for forty-five minutes. I finally figured out that it's chemo. "Don't start IV; stay away from me. Body doesn't want it." Or I didn't want it—that's for sure. And for several days after, my arm bending back as far as it can, thinking about it now makes my arm want to flex backwards.

Last week for the first time I began talking. Lots of talking, actually more like yelling. I have talked to Lila, but never impulsively lashed out physically and verbally during a session. Anger poured out regarding chemo. "Stop! Stop! Stop! Don't...Get away from me! Don't let them! Run! Run! They'll try to kill you! How can they do this to people? They shouldn't treat people this way!"

On my stomach, my head bent back, legs arching up, hands holding ankles. Back to the hog-tied thing.

"Have you ever been tied up like this?"

"No, this is totally bizarre."

"Have you ever been emotionally tied up like this?"

Billboard time! Total clarity! This is how I felt each time I went to chemo. "Get away from me, you SOB, I'll kill you—don't think I won't!" I spent the rest of the session bad mouthing all the kind souls who had helped me at Stanford. Phew. I'm so glad I won't walk around the rest of my life with that churning around inside. I can't believe it was even there.

Now I know what triggered cancer. Our whole church-split disaster that occurred seven years ago. We had attended this church since we were married. The congregation was truly one big family, that is, until the pastor got on the wrong path and tried to establish a dictatorship. We all struggled and agonized until finally things got so bad that many families in desperation left the church. We were one of the families to leave. It felt like a divorce. The split was more traumatic than I ever dreamed possible. It was the first occasion of insomnia for me. I initially went five days with no sleep, and it took nine months until I slept normally again. It was my introduction to sleeping pills.

Yesterday in cranial, I experienced a feeling so huge, like a balloon being blown up in my abdomen until I felt like I would pop. "Oh my gosh, I don't know what it is. It hurts!" I was near panic; the pain was steadily increasing.

Lila was quietly urging, "Look deeper." Praying, praying, Wham! Then a feeling like I was trying to vomit out all the turmoil, hurt, and pain of that church split. And during the disgust, the billboard, the absolute clarity of thought, "The stress of that church split is what triggered the cancer." The stress involved in that whole fiasco is what caused my body to misfire. And immediately after understanding what caused the cancer to begin, I thought, "Am I done now? Done with this whole healing process of unraveling all this stinky stuff from my life? Is it finally over?"

Rick in bed, feeling sick with serious head and chest pain. Lying next to him, feeling huge energy flowing from his head. He is obviously in a huge amount of discomfort and pain when he suddenly bolts up to a sitting position, arms in front of his chest, hands curled in, looking crippled. "I couldn't help you, I couldn't save you!" he yells. "I wanted to take the medicine for you, but I couldn't! I couldn't do anything to save you. I was helpless!" The dam has finally broken. Sitting on the bed sobbing, my husband finally releases the fear and anxiety of cancer. I haven't seen him cry since the stove in the back of the truck incident. One year of frustration and fear, and he never cried.

I'm so relieved, so thankful. "Cry, Honey, cry. Let it out, let it all out. Don't lug that stuff around anymore!"

He later told me that when he sat up on the side of the bed, his hands felt like a million needles were poking his hands. They hurt so bad, he couldn't move them. That was how my hands and feet had felt during chemo.

I'm in complete and total awe and wonder at God's faithfulness, mercy, and grace. We have spent the last five days watching all the walls between us crumble and fall. Walls we didn't even know existed. We are totally free now, and it's beyond imagination. Free to love without inhibitions, fears, resentments, questions. Pure, free-flowing love.

It turns out that God has had us on a path to this point, I suppose our whole life. Now that Rick has been selling properties the last three years, all decreasing his stress level significantly, he says that he felt like he was carrying a huge cement ball around three years ago and staggering under the weight. Selling each property was a small piece of the ball off his back. Then last week the big cancer explosion. And now the ball is gone, leaving us totally free and unencumbered in our love.

This last month has been life changing. God is working full time with us. Rick has released cancer fears, anxieties, and realized the depth of unfelt emotions and stress he had stashed away for thirty years. He has struggled greatly and is working so hard to get through this. He says it's the hardest thing he has ever done.

We do craniosacral every night, sometimes until 2 or 3 in the morning, releasing, agonizing, and processing buried emotions. Painful. Excruciating. Reminding him it will come off in layers, "Let your body work through each layer as it comes. I know it's uncomfortable. Awful to feel those feelings again. Work through them, release, never to be felt again. No longer stored somewhere to cause pain, anxiety, anger, illness. Let it out." Unbelievably intense.

Issues in our lives that I once considered tiny creeks . . . now we are uncovering the river that fed the creek, and then the stream that fed the river, and the lake that fed the stream. So many issues are intertwined and connected. We pump the lakes dry one by one. Angers, hurts, fears from as far back as our dating days. Looking back, we could understand how and why we had reacted the way we did and see how those early days had set us up for the weak areas in our marriage. Unearthing and reevaluating them is now creating total freedom.

I was anxious to attend the next CST class in San Francisco. The first morning we are asked to introduce ourselves and briefly explain how we got here. How I got here. Who would even believe this story? What part do I tell? What's the best way to briefly summarize what this whole process of CST has meant to me? I am deep in prayer as my turn draws near. I stand. "Good morning! My name is Sandy Howard. I went to cranial a couple years ago during a very stressful time in my life. I always thought energy stuff was for whackos, but God brought me to a point of desperation in my life a year and a half ago where I was open to try something very different.

Craniosacral Therapy, simply, saved my life. Through the treatments, God healed me from wounds I was aware of and wounds I didn't even know I had. I had no idea my body had stored trauma, emotional and physical trauma, and that my mind and body were so interconnected.

I've been working on my husband for the past year and a half, doing massage and CST, and just last month, he finally "got it," finally started releasing his own trauma. Now that he has experienced it, he understands how God used this whole process to heal me. In fact, he and my mom are next door right now in the CST I class." I sat down to a rousing applause.

Rick would share with his class that weekend how CST had healed his painful heel. He had been limping around during most of my treatment and couldn't find any relief. I had been doing cranial with him for a while, but the heel still hurt. He finally bought some of those expensive inserts and a first-class work boot. Seven hundred dollars later, the heel still hurt. But after his cancer blowout, where he relived how frustrated he had been during my treatment and his intense frustration that he could not take the medicine for me, his heel stopped hurting. It has not bothered him since.

I know God could have healed my emotional trauma in an instant. I know there are many other modalities that He works through to heal people every day. But CST was the path He gave me for healing. Just as He provided the amazing people at Stanford for my physical healing, so He provided Lila and CST for my emotional healing. And I am so very thankful for both.

When Joel was on the swim team, he experienced a very challenging season. This particular season he went from dominating every race to losing every race. It was not because of anything he had done differently. Simply, the other boys matured into men. Skinny competitors were suddenly rippling with muscles and shaving, while our stick boy had grown a couple inches but was skinnier than ever. He ended up tying for league champion in his division, a huge lesson for him in perseverance and the reward of plain old hard work.

During his season of trial, it was easy to tell Joel he had to be patient, keep working hard, and persevere through the swim season. "In the end, God will honor your faithfulness." It was easy to sit back, nod our heads, and think how difficult times will make him a better person, better equipped for life. Little did we know that God had a perseverance plan for our entire family. Because difficult times truly do make us better people, better equipped for life. Through trials, we learn that what counts is not the prize at the end of the journey but how we run the race.

I look inside and see changed attitudes and personal growth and know that God has brought us many, many miles these last two years. And now I am truly thankful for the blessing of cancer. It has given us an incredible opportunity to truly understand how short this life is and how important it is to live out the time we're given with purpose. We all have an inner power, a jet engine, that strains to pull us in the direction God desires, and we will never find perfect peace until we follow. There were many days I thought I wouldn't live, and some days I wished I hadn't. In this pit, I learned to learn the lesson the teacher has for me, rather than resenting the teacher. I'm learning that the more I let God take me over, the more truly myself I become—because He made me. I'm learning not to live in the past or worry about the future, but to trust what I cannot see more than what I can. And on the other side of cancer, life becomes an expression of gratitude.

But the battle never ends. I had my quarterly check up last month. Dr. Carmon palpated my breasts and stepped back in satisfaction. Everything's fine so far. . . His mutt gets a turn. Cool, so far, so good. Dr. Denis's mutt is next. Uh, huh, we're almost done here. Dr. Denis steps forward, the drumming fingers start their incessant, methodical journey from the base to the top, but at the top he stops . . . backs up, palpates again . . . stops, backs up . . . my heart has stopped. I want to hit him. I take a deep breath and brave a look in his eyes. "Alright, Fred, what have you got?"

"Well, I just feel a small lump here . . . have you felt this one?"

Sure enough, there it is, and it's long and oval shaped like my original tumor. I truly am confident that the cancer is gone, that it will not come back. My body has been purged of all negative emotions and all past traumas are completely erased, processed, given to God. Rick and I help each other on a weekly basis to rid ourselves of the stuff that accumulates with daily life, and we both make an effort not to store any negative emotions. Something negative happens, negative person spews our way, and we consciously process the content and very deliberately hand it off to God. "Do not carry anything."

And yet when this dear man says, "Have you felt this?" I have to will my body to breathe, "Don't slide down that slope of fear. God is in control." He's proven Himself so faithful, so why do I so easily slide down the slippery slope? We know the massive radiation doses cause tissue changes for up to three years. We've had a scare at every single follow-up appointment but one, and they end up being just that. Just a scare. Benign tissue. Just a jolt to keep me focused on what's important in life. In fact, Rick related how the previous visits scare . . . "What's this? Was this here before?" Followed by ultrasound to the site revealing the beautifully benign tissue . . . all had him unsettled until God reminded him He was truly in control.

Rick needed a replacement window for a rental that day, an odd size, and had just measured the window that morning. He drove uptown past a yard sale and voila! Propped against the house is a funky-sized window, which, of course, was the exact size he needed. He drove back to the rental, popped the window in, and done. God was telling him, "Look, I can handle this. I care about all the details of your life. How much more do I care about your wife! Don't allow yourself to slide into fear. Stake a post on the top of the slope, and hold on!"

I know some of you would just consider that luck. We don't. Back in the exam room, I was full of confidence. "It's near the original scar site, the area that got blasted by radiation."

"I'll just keep my eye on it until my next appointment; and if it's changed, we can ultrasound it then."

"Alright," Dr. Denis agrees, "if that's how you want to do it."

We leave the hospital in a puff of confidence. So we're going to face these scares every three months for a few more years until my tissues are done shifting. We can handle this. Back home I experience sharp pain in my left rib cage. The same spot that was the home of my original Texas-sized fear, the one that kept me from sleeping for so long, the same spot where I feared for Bryce's health. As Rick gently places his hand on my rib and directs his beautiful energy my way, billboard time, I realize I'm afraid cancer has returned. Hugely afraid. I walk to the phone and make the appointment for the ultrasound. A week later, the radiologist guides the ultrasound wand over the new lump and my breast is illuminated on her screen. The three of us stare intently at the blur. "This is all tissue, she explains."

"What's that dark border?" Rick asks.

"Oh, that's the muscle around your lung." Five minutes of intense scrutiny.

"Do you see anything?"

"No, it all appears to be healthy tissue. No cysts or tumors show up!"

I hop off the table and suck in a huge lungful of thanksgiving. Just another false alarm. Trina's cute Irish brogue on the message machine, "Sandy, Dr. Denis confirms the negative ultrasound, but he would still like for you to schedule a needle aspiration of that site just to make sure." We look at each other in amazement. Will it ever end?

No, it never will. That's part of being a survivor and the blessing of the continual unknown that forces us to live by faith. Because when the earth moves . . . I look up.